W9-DJA-743

THE *New* DIABETES WITHOUT FEAR

DR. JOSEPH I. GOODMAN
with W. WATTS BIGGERS

AVON BOOKS ◆ NEW YORK

The authors gratefully acknowledge permission to include material from the following:

From "A Dialogue About Diabetes and Exercise" by E.A. and D.F. Sims. Reprinted from *Diabetes Forecast*. Copyright © 1974 by permission of the American Diabetes Association.

From "Juvenile Diabetes: A Tragic Difference in Children" by B. Vincent, *The Cleveland Press*, May 22, 1974. Copyright © 1974. By permission of *The Cleveland Press*.

From "Life With Diabetes" by L. Matthews and E. Hill, *Diabetes Newsletter*, Diabetes Association of Greater Cleveland, 2022 Lee Road, Cleveland, Ohio 44118, April, 1974. By permission of *Diabetes Newsletter*.

From "Ron Santo and Diabetes: Accepted It, Live a Full Life" by J. Shaw. Reprinted from *Sportsmedicine* Magazine, June 1974 by permission of the publisher, McGraw-Hill, Inc.

THE NEW DIABETES WITHOUT FEAR is an original publication of Avon Books. This edition has never before appeared in book form.

AVON BOOKS
A division of
The Hearst Corporation
1350 Avenue of the Americas
New York, New York 10019

First Avon Books Printing: July 1995

THE FACTS

- There are over 14 million Americans with diabetes.

- Much of the drama and tragedy we see in movies and on TV that relates to diabetes is either untrue or preventable.

- Every diabetic has an individual insulin dosage that is best for him or her.

- Today, oral drugs are used successfully by nearly one-third of all diabetic patients.

- The celebrity roster of people with diabetes includes superstars in the worlds of sports, dance, movies, theater and television.

- Diabetics can—and do!—lead full, active, healthy, successful lives.

CONTENTS

v

FOREWORD

WHAT A WONDERFUL time to update Dr. Goodman's book. Fifteen years after the publication of *Diabetes Without Fear*, the results of the first long-term diabetes-care study, the Diabetes Control and Complications Trial (DCCT), have been released, and the findings confirm the premise of Dr. Goodman's book. This ten-year research project, financed by the National Institute of Diabetes and Digestive and Kidney Diseases and conducted at twenty-nine medical centers in the United States and Canada, showed definitively that despite the avalanche of gloom-and-doom predictions to the contrary, *diabetics who are willing to give their condition proper care can live long and healthy lives, free from the complications commonly considered to accompany diabetes, or with only minimal effects from them.* By keeping good control of their disease—taking frequent tests of their blood-glucose level and working closely with their medical teams—diabetics in the study were able to reduce the onset of serious complications by an average of 50–60 percent! Some were even able to *reverse* mild kidney disease.

"The discovery of insulin was an absolute miracle," says Dr. Phillip Gorden, speaking for the DCCT, "and this study is in the ballpark of comparison."

There is a second important reason for revising and reissuing *Diabetes Without Fear*. Thanks to major technical advances made over the past fifteen years, proper diabetic care has become far, far easier. The small, portable, easy-to-use yet highly reliable machine for measuring blood sugar is the most remarkable example.

But given such advances plus the confirming research of the DCCT study, is there still a *need* for this book? Will the newly diagnosed diabetic continue to be burdened with dire predictions? Will the gloom-and-doom announcements go on? Will the focus on fear of both the disease and its control (insulin) continue? Unfortunately, the answer appears to be a very definite yes. Although the results of the DCCT cannot be ignored, they are not likely to change the behavior and attitude of the vast number of doctors, nurses and other health-care workers who induce diabetic neurosis in patients and their families because they believe that proper diabetic care is best assured through emphasis on the horrors of failure rather than the benefits of success.

Nor is much likely to change the tone of those brochures designed to solicit funds for diabetes research, brochures sent regularly by organizations in need of financial support. Invariably, they focus on the most negative aspects of the disease. For example, a letter for the 1994 Annual Fund Drive of the Diabetic Action Research and Education Foundation declares:

I'm confident we can cure through research America's dreaded major cause of new blindness, major cause of amputation, major cause of kidney failure. I'm talking about DIABETES, the disease that will, this year alone, cause 12,000 cases of new blindness, will kill 10,000 by kidney failure, will result in more than 50,000 lower extremity amputations, will kill about 150,000 American people. . . . Diabetes is draining. It is relentless. And all we can do today is treat the symptoms by cutting off limbs, giving multiple insulin shots daily, attempting to restore eyesight through laser surgery, providing kidney dialysis treatments . . . but NO CURE.

Notice the inevitability so pronounced in this statement. Nowhere is there any reference to the fact that the diabetic has some say as to whether or not blindness or kidney failure or amputation will be the end result of the diabetes. Nowhere is there any suggestion that care resulting in "controlled" versus "uncontrolled" diabetes will affect the outcome. Such material gives the distorted impression that a diabetic has little chance of living a normal life—and there are far too few books out there to offset this neurosis-building negativity. Yes, this is the perfect time to update and release this book.

W. Watts Biggers, 1994

THE *New*
DIABETES
WITHOUT
FEAR

1

FICTION VERSUS FACT

"THE MOST AMAZING thing about diabetes is the complete lack of true knowledge that exists about it," says Mary Tyler Moore. "When I first learned I had it, I was very frightened. I wondered, 'Am I going to be an invalid? Will I be bedridden?' I just didn't know."

Unfortunately, the actress's experience is not unusual. Diabetes is probably the most misunderstood of all diseases—so much so that by the time the majority of my patients come to consult me for advice on the management of their diabetes, they have already developed emotionally crippling inhibitions which prevent them from enjoying the normal existence that should be theirs.

The news that one has an incurable disease—*any* incurable disease—is traumatic in itself, and in the case of diabetes, what the typical patient knows of the disease only serves to magnify the trauma. Thanks to pseudoscientific books, so-called documentaries on television and old wives' tales, the newly diagnosed patient quickly develops a swarm of unrealistic fears about diabetes. The disease is connected with visions of physical deterioration, shock from too much insulin and coma from too *little* insulin, gangrene, amputation, blindness and other dangerous complications. The diabetic worries about gainful employment, about the possibility of having children or even entering into marriage. Another type of fear and frustration arises with the thought of dietary restrictions and the inability to have sugar or alcohol ever again. The list of frightening apparations is endless.

In addition to the terrible toll such unnecessary fears take on the patients themselves is the heavy burden they place on members of the diabetic's family. Husbands and wives of diabetics wonder if their marriages can ever be "normal" again. Brothers and sisters of diabetics, often neglected in favor of the overprotected diabetic child, are often forced into a confused, guilt-ridden existence. Children of diabetics develop unhealthy eating habits and doubts about their futures. Parents of diabetics often feel plagued by gnawing guilt, blame themselves for their child's fate and doubt their ability to cope with the future.

"I honestly wasn't too upset when they first told me my son had it," said Keith, a hospital worker. "I'd seen lots of diabetics in my job. But then I remembered this TV story—a police show— about a diabetic who went into a coma just because he accidentally took too much insulin without eating. And then I remembered I'd heard the same thing from a neighbor, about how her nephew almost died from it. And right away I got to wondering what it was going to be like worrying every day about being certain we did everything just right for my son and whether something terrible would happen to him. All of a sudden I didn't think I could handle it. I started to fall apart.''

All too often, television programs that mention diabetes and/or insulin do so in the most negative context possible. For example, a recent episode of ''Emergency 911'' opened with a woman slumped over the steering wheel of her car as it rolled downhill. And host-narrator William Shatner informed viewers, ''The police first thought the driver was a diabetic who had gone into an insulin coma.'' Only much later did Shatner explain that the woman had actually been an epileptic! Another recent example occurred in December 1993, on the popular ''Unsolved Mysteries'' series. Here the episode focused on a nurse who injected insulin into the intravenous bags of two patients in order to murder them.

Consider how such stories affect newly diagnosed diabetics as they first learn that insulin must be self-injected on a daily basis! They might as well be told that their medication will be a daily dose of arsenic. No wonder so many diabetics and their families suffer tremendous mental anguish—not because of the reality of their disease, but because of unfounded fears about what they *believe* the disease and its control will be like, and what they believe the disease will do to them. I have invented a term for this dangerous emotional disturbance: *diabetic neurosis*. It is a vicious neurosis, often more destructive than the disease itself, and it usually begins the moment patients are told that they have diabetes. Why?

First of all, few people are prepared for the discovery that they have the disease. Although untreated diabetes has very recognizable symptoms—frequent urination, excessive thirst, insatiable hunger, weight loss, fatigue—most determinations are made well before such symptoms become severe; usually the diagnosis is made by chance, during a routine medical checkup by the patient's doctor, in a hospital where the patient has been admitted for some other disorder or even during a preemployment or insurance examination. Having had no previous suggestion of the illness, the typical patient is armed with nothing but inflammatory hearsay. Imagine, then, the reaction to the announcement that he or she has diabetes.

"It was like a building fell on me," Brian, a jewelry salesman in his mid-thirties, told me. "I've always been an active guy, and when the insurance doctor told me I had diabetes, it seemed like a dead end for my whole life. Maybe I didn't know too much about it, but what I did know was all bad."

Brian had always prided himself on his sound physical condition. He was an avid jogger. "When they told me about the diabetes, right away I thought about a book I'd read—this story about a guy who lost his legs—and that made me think about my own legs. I remember reaching down to touch them and wondering if the next thing would be that they'd have to chop them off."

Fear of complications is one of the primary causes of diabetic neurosis. Although the recently completed Diabetes Control and Complications Trial (DCCT) offers clear evidence that proper care of diabetes can allow the patient to lead a normal life, the strict, somewhat time-consuming regimen used by the controlled diabetics in the study tends to frighten away some newly diagnosed patients. "It doesn't sound like there'll be any time for anything but worrying about my sugar tests," a busy young advertising executive complained. "I don't think I can handle that. . . . I don't think I'll even try." And too many of those who talk about or write about the DCCT make it appear that a patient who refuses to practice this very strict "perfect" control might just as well practice no control at all.

Making matters still worse is the fact that diabetes requires that patients depend on a medicine, insulin, which frightens people almost as much as the disease itself. "I've heard things, you know," a dental receptionist told me. "Insulin shock, and all of that. From the minute they told me I had the disease, I've been worrying so much, I can't sleep right. And I'm afraid to take anything to make me sleep. My boss says that might not mix with insulin. So I'm becoming a nervous wreck. My doctor says if I don't calm myself down, I'm a prime candidate for ulcers."

The problem of the patient's lack of accurate information is often compounded by the physician's out-of-date or deliberately severe attitude toward the disease. In the case of a twenty-one-year-old college student named Mary, her gynecologist, discovering her diabetes in the course of a routine examination, immediately sat her down and volunteered this advice: "Since you have diabetes, you must carefully weigh the problems of marriage. You probably can't conceive. And if you do, there are all the dangers associated with pregnancy in diabetes—acidosis, hypertension and so on. If you should manage to overcome these hazards, the baby probably will not live.

If it does, it will most likely be afflicted with congenital deformities.''

An incredible diagnosis of the situation—totally untrue! Luckily, Mary was a very level-headed young woman. When she came to me, we were able to reapproach the subject, wipe away this misinformation, and send her on looking forward to a happy, well-rounded life, complete with husband and children. But imagine the psychological damage that might have been done to a patient with a less stable personality—one like twenty-three-year-old Darlene, for example.

This young woman was so fearful and guilt-ridden about her future that she insisted on attempting to cure herself through ''faith in God.'' Although her pastor and his wife, as well as her doctor, sought desperately to dissuade her from attempting this ''faith cure,'' the distraught young woman persisted. After three days without insulin, Darlene lapsed into a coma and needlessly, tragically died.

Or consider the case of David, the diabetic son of actress Dina Merrill, a leading actress of the sixties and a prominent socialite. Ms. Merrill explained why diabetic neurosis was responsible for her son's death: ''He was sure that his life would be short, or interfered with by blindness or something because of the diabetes, so he wanted instant results with everything, wanted to pack as much living in while he could. With him, it was always speed, speed, speed. Fast cars, fast boats. That's what killed him.''

David died in a high-speed motorboat accident just ten days short of his twenty-fourth birthday. What a tragic waste.

Yet even this was not the end of the story, as far

as diabetic neurosis was concerned. Convinced that diabetes was directly hereditary, Dina Merrill guiltily researched her family tree. "We've checked back on both sides of the family, but we haven't found it yet. Evidently it can skip five or six generations." The truth is, although we know that a person with diabetes is more likely to have other members of the family who are diabetic, there is no compelling evidence that diabetes is directly inherited.

Misinformation, then, is the chief cause of diabetic neurosis, a situation which is only worsened by most of the current literature.

"The more I read," says Brian, "the worse I feel. Diabetes sounds like the first step toward everything bad. Right away, you're stopped from eating and drinking anything you want, but that doesn't guarantee a thing. You don't live longer. It just *seems* longer. If you cut your foot, you may lose it. And if you just sit in a chair and watch TV, you'll probably go blind."

It's not difficult to locate some of the possible sources of Brian's unnecessarily gloomy understanding of diabetes. A recent fund-raising piece (May 17, 1993) from the highly respected Joslin Diabetes Center in Boston asks the reader for funds to help "ease the strain of living with diabetes" and offers these examples of the "desperate plight" of the diabetic and his or her family:

Although Bobby's parents try very hard to time his meals to his activities and make sure he takes his insulin regularly, his blood sugar is still difficult to control because artificially injected insulin just can't keep up with the body's own internal timing.

When 34-year-old Joe exercises, he often feels low when he really isn't and he eats extra food in a panic—causing his blood sugar to go even higher.

In an even more extreme case, little Lindsay, who takes her insulin faithfully, tries to watch for side effects like blurred vision, shaking or fatigue. But her intensive insulin treatment has impaired her body's ability to express hypoglycemia so, even though she *thinks* she's reducing her risk of diabetic complications, her insulin may be masking dangerous symptoms.

This type of desperately unbalanced statement, although made for the undeniably good cause of soliciting funds for research, clearly does more harm than good. Imagine the mental anguish of the newly diagnosed diabetic or a member of the family reading such a statement. Linda is an example. This is the letter she wrote to a very prestigious magazine after reading a special issue devoted to the "future" for diabetics: "I was terrified by your special issue. My own doctor tells me that I don't have anything to worry about with my eyes, yet your magazine says that most diabetics are going to lose their sight! What can I do to prevent this? What are my chances of going blind?"

Denise J. Bradley gets to the heart of the problem in her marvelous book *Sweet Recovery* (1992) when she points out that too many doctors and nurses fail to understand, or, at least, acknowledge that *con-*

trolled diabetes and *uncontrolled diabetes* are really two different diseases. "In the first," says Ms. Bradley,

> with a few adjustments in habits and life-styles, the diabetic will be "normal" in the sense that he can do the things normal people do and be healthy, maybe even more so because he has learned to observe changes in his body. With the other, uncontrolled diabetes, come the sickness, the side effects and the misery. For too long, I had been caught up in the vicious cycle of uncontrolled diabetes, not knowing my suffering was unnecessary. What a difference it made in my attitude to learn about my disease. Knowledge and hope were replacing my long-term fear and resignation.

Although the effects of diabetes obviously can be very serious and should not be minimized, the important fact is that diabetics can lead healthy, active lives; that persons who have had diabetes for twenty, thirty, forty, even fifty years can function quite normally; that today there are television and movie stars, high government officials, even professional sports figures with diabetes who lead full, highly successful lives without a hint of abnormality. In fact, because they take better care of themselves, their lives are perhaps longer and healthier than if they had *not* had diabetes.

In fact, in the view of the medical profession's majority, diabetes *cannot* be ranked with heart disease and cancer as a leading killer. Most doctors are inclined to view diabetes as a more-or-less benign process. In fact, Dr. L. Matthews of Case Western

Reserve University wrote, "I've had diabetes since 1957 . . . [and] if one *has* to have a chronic disease, and we really have no choice, then I feel we are fortunate to have diabetes."

But the average diabetic knows little of this. Everything he or she reads or hears about the disease is presented from the kind of pessimistic viewpoint that leads to such questions as: "Am I finished?" "Can I get married?" "Should I have children?" "Will I soon be too weak to hold a job?"

And while questions such as these are bombarding the brain, the diabetic can expect to be arbitrarily denied life and health insurance by some companies, rejected by misguided potential employers, even thwarted in any application for a driver's license.

The vice-president of a large corporation was eager to hire a very talented young woman who was one of my patients. During the preemployment examination, the company physician discovered that the applicant was a diabetic and stated, "Your sugar is high. I'll have to reject you." Despite a recommendation—a very strong one—from a company officer, the doctor refused my patient, labeling her as unsuitable for employment. You can imagine what this did to the patient's sense of purpose and self-confidence, and what a waste of talent it was—all due to private and professional ignorance about the true nature of diabetes when it is under control.

Some twenty years ago, when race car driver Dick Batchelder learned that he had diabetes, one of the first things he recalled was someone once telling him that diabetics often could not get a license to drive. "I thought of that and wondered, 'What happens to me now? What about my job, my family, my racing career?' " It was an oppressive fear of a type he had never known before. It almost conquered him, but he managed to break free, and that same year went on to set a new track record in the Canadian Classic at Star Speedway in New Hampshire.

There are hundreds of human success stories like Batchelder's. Consider these: sports greats Jonathan Hayes (football), Bill Talbert (tennis) and Bill Gullickson (baseball). New York City Ballet soloist Zippora Karz. Actors Mary Tyler Moore, Carol Channing, Wilford Brimley. "Diabetes is certainly not the worst thing I've ever known," says Brimley. "To tell you the truth, it's been kind of good—kind of exciting—to have this challenge in my life."

Why does the public so seldom see or hear positive thoughts like this about diabetes? Why, instead, are so many depressing words written on the subject?

If blindness is only a sometime result of diabetes, why do so many articles, books and television shows imply that it is inevitable?

If candy, cake and alcohol need not be dropped from the diabetic's diet, why do so many written materials state precisely the opposite?

If diabetic parents need not live in fear that their children are certain to be diabetic, too, why aren't they told this?

If the use of insulin can be simple and safe, why should movies and television shows imply the opposite?

Why, in short, has such a large percentage of writing about diabetes focused on the most negative aspects of the disease?

Certainly much of what is being disseminated was once true—but is true no longer. Certainly, too, there is far more drama, far more sales appeal, in a story that builds to tragedy—to gangrene, amputation, divorce, blindness, frustration, coma, death—than one in which all ends well. Perhaps those doing the writing have been so concerned with the importance of following prescribed treatment that they have neglected the positive aspects of diabetes.

Regardless of the reason, the fact is that very little has been written about the great strides medicine has made in understanding diabetes and in helping patients live with it easily, safely and comfortably. And tragically, this vacuum, combined with a growing mountain of misinformation, has served only to insure that diabetics and their families suffer from diabetic neurosis. It is a mountain I have had to confront again and again throughout my more than fifty years as a diabetes specialist, in both private and hospital practice.

Today, there are an estimated fourteen million Americans who have diabetes, and, conservatively, another forty million whose lives are intimately intertwined with that of someone who is a diabetic. Thus, a tremendous percentage of this nation's total population is affected by a myriad of completely unnecessary emotional disturbances connected with this disease. This makes diabetic neurosis one of the most serious health problems facing our country.

In this book, I discuss the various fears and anxieties which preoccupy the diabetic and his family, frequently drawing on patients' own words and analyzing in some detail the background of their emotional reactions. I have undertaken to counteract these disturbing factors in much the same way that I do in my private practice: I present all sides of the problem under discussion from a rational scientific standpoint, substituting medical realities plus sound, practical advice and how-to information for exaggerations and half-truths. In this way, I offer the diabetic patient and members of the family a way to view their circumstances with reassurance and optimism—and realistic hope for a normal life.

2
BASIC QUESTIONS AND ANSWERS ON DIABETES

IF IGNORANCE AND misinformation are the basis for diabetic neurosis, then education is obviously the key to prevention and cure. But what kind of education? How much? And how should it be obtained?

"I honestly think my doctor's attitude changed toward me the minute he found out I had diabetes," a thirty-five-year-old computer operator told me. "He always took plenty of time with me before, but when I got diabetes, he just handed me a pamphlet from some clinic and told me to talk with his nurse."

How much time should the doctor spend explaining the nature and treatment of diabetes? Physicians sometimes turn their patients over to nurses or dieticians or even other diabetics, but this is not necessarily the best possible schooling. There is, after all, a great deal that is new and very meaningful for the diabetic and the family to learn. While most of it may seem quite simple to a thoroughly trained physician, this is not likely to be the case for patients and their families.

''More than anything else, it's the needle that frightens me,'' a young mother told me. ''I'm always afraid it will break or bend while I'm giving myself the shot, so I hate the idea of being alone when I do it. And yet I don't like my husband or my children—especially my children—watching me. So I keep on doing it alone, even though I'm terrified.''

Fear of the needle breaking or bending is only one of many fears expressed to me by patients who have not been properly educated about diabetes. Typical questions are:

What about air bubbles? Is it true they can kill?

Will my arms and legs become unsightly in the places where the needles are constantly used?

Would there be less chance of this if I have fewer shots per day?

If some of the insulin runs out, should I try to give myself a small second shot, or could that be dangerous?

Are some insulins better than others?

Is it dangerous for diabetics to exercise? Should I stop my child from participating in school sports?

It is time to offer some answers.

Who should educate?

From the moment diabetes is diagnosed, both the patient and the family should enter a learning process sufficient to dispel the rumors, myths and distortions associated with diabetes, but also to make the diabetic's ''tools''—diets, exercise regimen, insulin, needles or medication—as familiar and user-friendly as the controls of an automobile are to a skilled driver.

The new diabetic requires a bare minimum of

twelve hours' of intense, individual instruction—but some physicians, perhaps considering themselves poor communicators or feeling they cannot economically devote this amount of time to the disease, do not undertake the instruction themselves but instead seek other methods for educating their patients.

Dr. B. R. Boshell, for example, was one of the first to maintain that other diabetics are the best teachers for new diabetic patients, and therefore turned over much of the responsibility for instruction to them. In this way, patients were taught how to estimate food exchanges at home or in restaurants, how to alter dosages of insulin and how to test for blood sugar. This instruction was supplemented by written material, including a handbook and an individualized "blue book" containing the patient's medication schedule and all tests from the first day of admission. There was also a "yellow book" for permanent recording of four-times-daily blood-sugar tests in the hospital and, later, at home.

Despite the arguable efficacy of these materials, however, I consider the process ineffective and even dangerous. First, the lack of formal training for such diabetes "teachers" tends to lower the level of importance attached to this education by new diabetics. If it were *really* important, they are inclined to think, my doctor would be doing this for me. Second, the patient-teachers may well be asked to respond to questions for which they are not properly prepared. Third, any errors these patient-teachers may themselves have picked up will be passed along and very likely compounded by their pupils.

Recognizing these dangers, some doctors have turned to courses offered by well-established units of specially trained personnel, such as nurses and dieticians and other "educators" (the American Association of Diabetic Educators [AADE] is an organization with several thousand members, many of them diabetics, and many of them "certified," which means they have passed an exam given by the association). But allowing newly diagnosed patients to obtain their knowledge about diabetic care through courses given by such educators also has intrinsic weaknesses. Consider the results of such a course offered at the E. J. Meyer Memorial Hospital in Buffalo, New York. Immediately following the course, the new patients appeared highly proficient at techniques such as insulin injection, but only three months later, both their general knowledge of the disease and their proficiency at self-care had declined decisively. Moreover, their course suffered a tremendously high dropout rate—of the original forty-six patients, only nine remained to complete the instruction.

The dropout rate was lower when offered to a second group, comprised of clinic outpatients; however, at the end of the program, their response to questions designed to test their knowledge of the management of diabetes was an average of only 55 percent correct. They had poor knowledge of meal planning and proper diet, and little idea of how to manage proper testing for acetone in the urine.

Nevertheless, doctor substitutes are often successful in the education of patients. What is too often overlooked or ignored is the fact that with diabetes, unlike most other diseases, education is not a subordinate matter in terms of patient health; rather, it is a *major* part of the "treatment." As such, it demands the physician's personal attention. Only in this way will the patient attach sufficient importance to the matter to listen and learn to the best of his or her ability, to stay until the "course" is complete and to receive the kind of answers their questions deserve.

In my view, the best service performed by nurses and dieticians and others who "educate" in this field is not the immediate instruction of diabetics on how the disease is to be treated; rather, it is the *implementation* of the instruction as supplied by the physician. It was in this capacity that nurses and dieticians were so successful in the recently completed Diabetes Control and Complications Trial.

Patient support groups are a different matter, of course. Members of such groups can be very helpful for the new patient in terms of keeping up motivation, offering examples which "prove it can be done" and opening up new lines of inquiry. Even here, however, newly diagnosed diabetics must be made to understand that innovations offered by members of a support group—new diets or exercises or combinations of insulin, and so on—are not to be traded like recipes at a baking convention. Any significant change in regimen must be checked out fully with the patient's own physician.

With diabetes, the relationship between patient and doctor is far more important than with many other diseases. Without respect and trust, the patient cannot be expected to treat the physician's orders with the proper sense of urgency, nor can the patient be expected to be truthful, especially since this sometimes demands embarrassing admissions. In the book, *Diabetes: A Guide to Living Well*, the authors write: "You have the right to choose a physician with whom you have a mutually rewarding relationship.

You need not feel guilty if you decide to change doctors because you want a better relationship.'' I would go further and say the diabetic not only has a *right* to choose the proper physician; he or she has a *duty* to do so. In making this choice, diabetics are choosing their future—healthy or unhealthy, controlled or uncontrolled. It is diabetics' duty to themselves and their families to make absolutely certain there is complete trust and respect for the physician selected.

What is diabetes?

The full name of the disorder is Diabetes Mellitus, and it results when the beta cells of the pancreas fail to provide a sufficient supply of effective insulin, causing excessively high levels of glucose in the blood. Without insulin, the body is unable to change foods—proteins, fats and carbohydrates—into the energy needed to sustain life and keep the body functioning properly, leading to weight loss and fatigue. We do not know precisely *why* this occurs, *why* the pancreas ceases to fulfill its insulin function, but age and obesity often play a role.

There are two basic types of diabetes.

- *Type 1:* (also called juvenile diabetes or IDDM—Insulin Dependent Diabetes Mellitus) An estimated 1.4 million Americans have Type 1 diabetes. Generally occurring in children or young adults, it affects more males than females and develops rapidly. The pancreas provides no insulin or very, very little, so that the patient is dependent upon injections of insulin for proper body function.

- *Type 2:* (also called NDDM—Noninsulin Dependent Diabetes Mellitus) An estimated thirteen million Americans have Type 2 diabetes which develops gradually. In Type 2, the pancreas does produce insulin, but the body resists using it properly, which means that greater amounts of insulin are needed to keep normal levels of glucose in the blood.

There is no known cure for diabetes, but it can be controlled in one of three ways, or by a combination thereof.

1. Diet and exercise
2. Oral medication
3. Insulin

Insulin

What is insulin?

On January 11, 1922, Drs. Frederick Banting and Charles Best injected an extract from an animal pancreas into the body of a teenager, Leonard Thompson, who lay gravely ill with diabetes. Almost immediately, Thompson improved, and within days of having been on the verge of death, the young man, whose weight had dropped to seventy-five pounds, had dramatically regained his weight and strength.

And so the world hailed the discovery of the extract, insulin, the first effective means of treating diabetes. It was a medical miracle, a momentous discovery, which eventually won a Nobel Prize for

Drs. Banting and Best. There is no way to overestimate the importance of their discovery. Without it, a book such as this one would be impossible, for there would be little to discuss on the positive side of diabetes for the millions who can now look forward to a happy, normal life.

Today, more than seventy years after Banting and Best's discovery, physicians have a wide variety of insulins to choose from for their patients, depending upon the source, the action time and the concentration.

The source

"Source" refers to where the insulin comes from. The original product was extracted from the pancreas glands of cattle or swine. These beef and pork insulins are still very much in use (sometimes in combination), but there is now an important third source, and it provides insulin identical to that produced by the human body. Commonly referred to as "human insulin," it was developed after scientists learned how to introduce recombined forms of the genetic material DNA (dioxyribonueleic acid) into bacteria, thereby permitting the protein-manufacturing portion of the bacteria to be programmed to produce human insulin. The product was first approved for clinical use in 1982.

Although for the most part insulin is insulin, there *are* some differences. The human body is designed to use *human* insulin, and it recognizes the difference between that and insulin produced by cattle or swine. So when beef or pork insulin is injected, the human body manufactures antibodies that quickly attack this foreign product. This means that a small amount of the beef or pork insulin will be tied up in the battle with the antibodies and is unavailable to work to lower blood sugar. Since this is not true for human insulin, it is likely that less of the latter will be needed for patient control. Thus, the insulins are not interchangeable, and this should be borne in mind in case a change is demanded, as is sometimes the case when a patient develops an allergic reaction to pork or beef insulin.

The action time

"Regular insulin," the original product produced by Banting and Best, works for a relatively short time, and it was primarily in order to prolong this period that other insulins were developed.

The following summary indicates the variety of preparations available. A given preparation is prescribed depending upon how long the doctor wishes the preparation to continue acting. Bear in mind that although various types are grouped together, *no substitutions should be made in any patient's program without the physician's approval.*

1. Short or rapid-acting insulins
   a. Regular
   b. Semilente
2. Intermediate-acting insulins
   a. 70/30
   b. NPH
   c. Lente
3. Long-acting insulins
   a. Ultra-lente
   b. PZI

Length of action time varies from one-half hour to thirty-six hours.

The concentration

"What about the different numbers on the insulin? My druggist was out of U-100 and offered to sell me U-40. I said no, and went shopping elsewhere, but it left me wondering."

Unless they have been given a thorough grounding in the diabetic "tools," patient and family alike are almost certain to be confused by the different concentrations of insulin available—U-100 versus U-40. In the case in question, the patient used better judgment than the druggist. Although in theory there is no reason why a patient using U-100 insulin could not substitute U-40, danger lies in possible miscalculation of the patient's prescribed dosage.

When it comes to insulin concentrations, all a patient and the family really need do is follow one basic rule: always keep sufficient insulin of the proper concentration on hand—always have one bottle in reserve—so that if your druggist is out of what you need, there is ample time for him to order more or you to shop at another drugstore. For those who wish to understand the differences between the concentrations of insulin, however, I will explain.

Not long ago, insulin was sold in three main concentrations: U-40, U-80, U-100. Today, only two of these are commonly prescribed—U-40 and U-100—and U-40 is continued only for patients for whom such low dosages are prescribed that U-100 would be difficult to measure. The difference in these preparations is how much liquid volume is contained for each unit of insulin—or, to put at it another way, how "pure" the preparation is in terms of insulin. With U-100 preparations, a single cubic centimeter (cc) of the liquid contains 100 units of insulin, while with U-40, that same amount of liquid contains only 40 units of insulin. Thus, you have to inject more than twice as much U-40 to get the same amount of insulin as with U-100.

Over the years, there has been much confusion because of the different concentrations. At one time, insulin syringes were marked with two scales, so that they could be used with either U-40 or U-80 insulin, and as a result, it was not uncommon for patients mistakenly to use the wrong scale and inject themselves with half—or, much worse—twice their prescribed dosage. The result in the latter case was often insulin shock. Today, as I've noted, insulin is commonly prescribed in only two concentrations—U-40 and U-100—and the syringes, which now contain only a single scale, are color-coded to match the color on the insulin bottles: U-40 is red, and U-100 is orange. Whenever practical, U-100 is recommended, especially because of its compatibility with our decimal system. And there is no danger if a doctor shifts a patient from U-40 to the more highly purified U-100 product. No actual change in insulin dosage is required, just a reduction in liquid volume, so diabetic control is unaffected. If a patient is in good control before the change, he or she should remain in good control afterward.

Other common concerns

Many patients fear needles and worry that there will be problems with their breaking or bending. However, needle quality today is excellent, and such fears are totally groundless. In my many years of practice, needle breaking or bending has never happened to one of my patients. Those concerned about the pain of needles might ask their doctors about jet injection. This special method of delivering insulin requires a separate prescription and is somewhat expensive, but it is covered by most medical insurance.

"It's an awful problem keeping my insulin refrigerated when I go to visit overnight. Is there any simple way to handle this?"

There certainly is: forget it. The complicated methods used by diabetics to insure refrigeration of insulin are totally unnecessary. I have talked with patients who carried ice or used special thermos bottles or other cold devices whenever they traveled for more than a day, but the truth of the matter is that although unopened bottles should be stored in the refrigerator, insulin being used by the patient does not deteriorate at room temperature and thus does not need refrigeration.

"I worry about air bubbles in the syringe. How dangerous are they? And if a bubble makes me lose any of the insulin, should I give myself a small second shot?"

Questions like these (and they are quite common) again point up the importance of proper patient education. A colleague told me recently of a patient who quite accidentally injected himself with a whole vial of air. Recognizing what he had done, the patient called for an ambulance and then lay down, prepared to die.

Actually, there is no danger from air—whether a

whole vial or a single bubble—unless it is injected directly into a vein. Air in the syringe is to be avoided because of this possibility, but the properly informed patient knows how unlikely this is, especially since he or she is trained to give injections in a manner that avoids the veins.

As for giving additional insulin if some should be lost (for whatever reason), the answer is an emphatic no. If the amount is relatively small, the loss may be ignored. If it appears to be more than a single unit or two, patients should consult their physician.

"A woman who lived in the neighborhood where I grew up had diabetes. She used to talk to my mother about it, and I will never forget those ugly places on her upper arms. I've been worried about this ever since they told me what my daughter has. I guess she'll have to get rid of all her short-sleeved blouses, won't she?"

This mother's fears for her daughter were groundless. The condition she referred to, lipoatrophy, never affected more than a relatively small percentage of diabetics at any time, and today even that number has been drastically reduced. Lipoatrophy—the appearance of hollowed-out areas at the site of frequent insulin injection—results from the disappearance of fat, and it is often preceded or accompanied by swelling (lipohypertrophy) in these same areas.

The cause of this was unknown until recently, and there was no specific treatment. Today, however, it is recognized that the condition is a reaction to certain material in insulin (noninsulin protein material and proinsulinlike substances) that produces antibodies. In 1973, the highly purified insulin U-100 was first introduced, and this has led to a marked decrease in the number of patients who display the allergic reactions that lead to lipoatrophy or lipohypertrophy. In fact, this new insulin has even proven effective in revitalizing the sunken or swollen areas of patients who had previously displayed these conditions. Dr. S. M. Wentworth and his associates, at a meeting of the American Diabetes Association in 1974, reported improvement or complete disappearance of atrophy due to insulin lipoatrophy in 85 percent of the patients tested, and similar results were reported for insulin allergy by a team from the Lilly Laboratory for Clinical Research.

One caution, however: although this purer insulin, U-100, has greatly reduced the incidence of unsightly tissue conditions, the diabetic is still well advised to rotate the site of insulin injections. Without such rotation, thickened skin may build up and make the giving of injections more difficult and uncomfortable. The following areas of the body are best for insulin injections, because they are at some distance from large blood vessels, joints and nerves:

- the upper, outer area of the arms
- the front and side areas of the thighs
- the buttocks
- just above the waist on the back
- the abdomen, except the area around the navel at the waistline

By methodically rotating these sites in a pattern designed with the help of a doctor or nurse, the patient avoids problems that might develop from repeated injection in a single area and also avoids using a spot that might still be tender from a previous injection.

Although purified insulin plus site rotation makes the occurrence of problems highly unlikely, patients should check the injection areas periodically, pressing gently and running fingertips across the skin. If lumps, knots or shallow areas are found or if there is pain or change of color at any injection site, this should be reported to the physician, and use of that area should be avoided until the matter has been fully discussed.

The best insulin dosage

"If I have diabetes because I lack adequate insulin, and if I inject adequate insulin, why don't I become completely normal?"

The answer is that, short of a transplant, medical science is unable to match the function of the pancreas. In order to make the diabetic completely "normal," insulin would have to be made available to the body at the precise times and in the precise amounts that it would be released from the pancreas of the nondiabetic person. And this cannot yet be done.

The diabetic whose pancreas is incapable of secreting sufficient insulin must rely on an injected product, one that is absorbed into the bloodstream at a uniform rate over several hours. The injected product cannot respond to body demands. For example, the regular rate of absorption will not increase because the patient decides to eat an especially heavy meal, nor will it decrease because the patient extends the hours between meals.

The simple truth is that, although insulin has been

available for almost three-quarters of a century, we are not yet skilled enough in its use to restore the blood sugar of the diabetic to absolute normal. Although I am confident this day will come in the not-too-distant future in one way or another, for the present, the proper treatment for the diabetic is that program that best enables his or her body to most closely approximate insulin normalcy on a consistent basis.

"Once my doctor decided on the right dosage for my diabetes, why should he change it? I had been doing fine for two months, and all of a sudden he changed the amounts. Does that make sense?"

Indeed it does. Be thankful that your doctor watches you carefully and notes the signs that indicate a need for change. Patients and their families should prepare themselves for an ever-changing pattern in terms of insulin dosage. Why? Because the blood glucose of diabetic patients is characteristically variable. Wide swings are commonplace. It is almost impossible to avoid such fluctuations even in the well-regulated diabetic.

It is a tragedy that great numbers of patients, having "managed" their diabetes by way of a fixed insulin dose over a period of many years, now suffer from crippling disabilities. Their blood-glucose levels have changed, but their insulin dosage has not. As the recent DCCT study has clearly confirmed, there is no rule more important to the insulin-taking diabetic than this one: frequent reassessment of the insulin dosage is essential.

"This guy and I were patients together at the hospital, and I know for a fact my blood sugar was never higher than his, but now that he's home he ends up taking only half as many injections as I do. Can you think of any logical reason for that?''

I certainly can. For one thing, the hospital environment and the home environment are quite different. Two patients might have similar blood-sugar patterns while in the hospital and quite different ones at home. More important, every patient is different, and requires an individualized dose. Moreover, patients should not complain about programs that require several doses of insulin. Some of the most common errors of treatment occur when physicians attempt to maintain diabetics on too few injections.

A classic example is one quoted by Dr. P. Forsham in connection with protamine zinc insulin. The arrival of this long-acting insulin back in 1946 was hailed as a great breakthrough. In one sense, this is true, but in another sense it was, in Dr. Forsham's words, ''the worst thing that ever could have happened to diabetes, because it failed to deliver the necessary big dose during peak body demand periods. Many juvenile diabetics who were on protamine zinc insulin exclusively for twenty years or more are now blind, sick and dying.''

There is no single foolproof method of fitting a patient's insulin dosage to the fluctuations that occur in his blood glucose level. About a multi-shot regimen versus those requiring only a single injection, Dr. Forsham says, ''Patients unaccustomed to multiple shots will complain at first but will soon feel so much better in the afternoon and evening that they will be happy to comply.''

Some years ago, Dr. Robert Jackson very successfully treated a large group of juvenile diabetics at the

University of Iowa, without complications, using four doses of regular insulin per day: morning, noon, at dinnertime and at bedtime. When the doctor suggested that an intermediate insulin might be substituted before dinner to avoid bothering the child for the late dose, the parents invariably asked, "Will my child get along as well on three doses of insulin as he has been doing on four?"

This attitude should be adopted by all patients. The question put to the doctor should not be: "How many shots can I get by with?" Rather, it should be: "How many shots will provide the best possible management of my diabetes?"

Insulin reaction

As we have mentioned, television and the movies have provided the American public with a steady diet of scary misinformation about common reactions to insulin, particularly hypoglycemia, or low blood sugar. What does hypoglycemia look and feel like? Here's a vivid description:

"Last week I had a horrible experience in school," an eighteen-year-old young woman relates.

"I knew something was wrong, so I went to the principal's office. I told the assistant principal I was feeling funny and needed orange juice. He went to the refrigerator and brought me some. Before I could drink it, I passed out, grabbed him and started pulling at him. Why do I always get violent when I have an insulin reaction? I want to hurt people. I make a damn fool of myself. I have only three more days of school, but I know the kids are talking. What do you think they're saying? By the way, I have a scholarship to college. Thank goodness I'm going to live away from home.''

In another case, that of a forty-five-year-old male, frequent periods of hypoglycemia often resulted in double vision, which made his wife and daughter fearful of letting him out of their sight. This, in turn, symbolized invalidism to this husband and father, making him feel old and dependent, and this ''loss of manhood'' in turn led to severe depression.

How is the diabetic to cope with hypoglycemia?

Normal functioning of the brain is dependent on an adequate supply of glucose and oxygen. If the blood-glucose level is allowed to become unduly low, the brain is unable to carry out its normal activity, and the body attempts to correct the problem by releasing chemicals called hormones that raise the blood-sugar level: glucagon, epinephrine and several others. Although these hormones help to raise blood-glucose levels, they also contribute to some very uncomfortable symptoms. Before the hormones have their effect, however, the low level of blood glucose affects the body's sympathetic nervous system, and the patient experiences symptoms that may include a rapid heart rate, pounding pulse, excessive perspiration, headache, hunger, pallor, nervousness, trembling, acute anxiety, abdominal pain, nausea, vomiting (on rare occasions) and blurred vision. If these first symptoms, the body's ''early warning system,'' go unheeded, the hormones released begin to add their effect, contributing to such symptoms as hyperexcitability, irritability, poor coordination, inability to concentrate, drowsiness, fatigue, confusion, inappropriate behavior, crying, loss of consciousness and generalized convulsions.

Such a listing of symptoms should make it clear that the violent conduct of the hypoglycemic highschool girl was not exceptional. The important point to bear in mind here is that forewarned should mean forearmed. With proper care and preparation, hypoglycemic symptoms need never develop; or, if they do, they can be counteracted in a matter of minutes or seconds.

Toward this end, schoolteachers and administrators should be given a thorough understanding of the symptoms, signs and treatment of insulin reactions, which may occur during school hours. Moreover, all diabetics, children and adults alike, should carry with them some source of sugar—honey or syrup or candy or even soda—which can be consumed at the first sign of insulin reaction.

A rapid, very neat way to treat such reactions is glucose gel. This thick, syrupy jelly is packaged in a collapsible tube for easy administration, and a generous squeeze releases the concentrated glucose into the patient's mouth. It is absorbed rapidly, and the hypoglycemia is overcome within fifteen to twenty minutes. Also available are glucose tablets (orange flavored), as well as other similar products. But the important point to bear in mind is not any particular type of sugar, but the fact that some form should always be carried by the diabetic.

In the nondiabetic, insulin secretion is regulated so that only the amount required at the present moment is released by the pancreas. When no longer needed, the flow of insulin into the bloodstream is shut off.

By contrast, the insulin administered to diabetic patients is not subject to the controls of the pancreas. The insulin dose is injected into the subcutaneous space (the area beneath the skin), where it remains until it is consumed, and during this period the insulin is absorbed into the bloodstream at a fixed rate. There is no shutoff valve. The insulin continues to lower the blood sugar even between meals, when the patient is without food. It is this situation which, if not understood and taken into account, can lead to hypoglycemia—when, for example, the patient's insulin dosage is based on the expectation of "snacking" every two hours and the snack is ignored—or, worse, when an entire meal is skipped.

Patients on low-calorie reducing diets are particularly prone to hypoglycemia unless extreme care is taken to reassess their insulin dosage on a regular basis. Many such overweight patients experience a complete reversal of their diabetes when they begin a low-calorie diet—often to such a degree that they begin to wonder if they ever had the disease. Obviously, a greatly reduced regimen of insulin is called for in patients on reducing diets. When the low-calorie diet is put into effect, insulin requirements may be lowered as much as 50 percent.

Another common cause of insulin reaction is more exercise than usual. No diabetic, young or old, needs to give up normal exercise or sports activity. He or she need only be properly prepared for what this exercise will demand. Physical activity revs up the body's metabolism, causing blood glucose to be consumed by the body at a more rapid rate, while the injected insulin continues to be absorbed by the body at the normal rate. The effect of this situation is graphically expressed by Dorothea Sims:

Early in my diabetes, I remember the sense of injustice with which I gulped orange juice laced with sugar during an insulin reaction which followed the unplanned-for and unrecognized exercise of running up-and-downstairs, looking after the children when they were sick all at once. I soon learned at a very basic level that, with my type of diabetes, I need to carry some form of sugar on me at all times, even in the most apparently routine situations such as cleaning house, shoveling snow or mowing the lawn.

Of course, this applies as well to the time when we plan a hike, a swim or a bike ride, or when I work in our vegetable garden. In these circumstances, I not only carry carbohydrate in some form with me, as well as my small insulin travel kit, but I always eat somewhat more than my usual intake at the meal before we begin, with emphasis on protein for its staying power—for example, an extra glass of milk and a cracker with peanut butter and jelly. I find that I need to supplement the meal with sugar about every twenty to thirty minutes when hiking or cross-country skiing.

In spite of years' of experience, there are still pitfalls for me. The commonest mistake is for me to forget to replenish the store of candy in my purse, parka or suitcase. If I am especially happy in some sort of exercise, I find that I have developed a kind of reflex yet subconscious method of evaluating all the elements in any given situation in order to stay up-to-date with the changing scene.

In my own head, I compare it to the skill with which we drive our cars, habitual enough so that it is not a distraction from work or play, and yet alert and calculating enough to respond to signs of imbalance.

Ms. Sims was entirely correct. Especially as they become more familiar with the signs and symptoms of their disease, diabetics need have no fear of hypoglycemia if they adhere to these few relatively simple rules:

1. Take special precautions with low-calorie diets; discuss any dietary change in detail with your physician.
2. When more than the usual amount of exercise is anticipated and the usual dosage of insulin injected, additional food must be consumed during and for several hours following the exercise.
3. Never go for long periods without food. Consume snacks in a manner that best coincides with the hours when your particular insulin regimen has its maximum effect—two to four hours for the short-acting insulins, six to eight hours for the intermediate insulins, twelve to sixteen hours for the prolonged insulins.
4. Snacks taken between meals or during exercise should be proteins or fats. The effect of carbohydrates in raising the blood sugar is not sufficiently prolonged to be an effective preventive. Fats and proteins, on the other hand, prolong

    the glycemic effect of food over a period of several hours.

5. Always carry with you some type of carbohydrate (such as sugar or candy) in case hypoglycemic symptoms occur.

6. Check your blood sugar level as often as possible, in accordance with your doctor's directions.

These rules, once thoroughly understood, can become as much a part of the diabetic's subconscious way of dealing with possible insulin reactions as the rules he or she learned in childhood about preventing colds. If this seems unrealistically positive, consider the case of the elderly lady who, after having taken insulin for many years, was told that her condition had improved to such a point that her insulin could be discontinued.

The woman was so accustomed to her daily care routine that she could not accept the diagnosis; she refused to be deprived of her insulin regimen, and in an attempt to have it reinstated, she insisted on needlessly checking her blood sugar several times before her next scheduled office visit. In addition, she insisted that eating without insulin might aggravate her diabetes. As a result, she curtailed her diet and lost several pounds, although previously she had been at her proper weight. It was necessary for her physician to prescribe a small dose of insulin daily as a placebo, after which she reverted to her previous, well-balanced state. In short, she had become so habituated to her set of rules that she could not do without them even when they were no longer necessary—clear evidence that the diabetic can become reconciled to (even happy with) the regimen.

The oral drugs

"Since our daughter doesn't like needles, couldn't we substitute one of the oral insulins?"

This is a commonly asked question, but I'm afraid there are no "oral insulins." Insulin can only be administered via injection. The oral antidiabetic drugs available today are not insulin but work in other ways to reduce high blood glucose. The oral drugs cannot help everyone, but for many diabetics they are, as one of my patients put it, "the answer to a prayer." I vividly recall the tremendous wave of enthusiasm that swept through the medical profession many years ago when the early reports on these drugs were presented. At one meeting, every seat in the auditorium was occupied, and some doctors, their dignified images notwithstanding, were almost literally hanging from the rafters in order to hear the presentation. Their hopes were not disappointed.

Many diabetics were taken off insulin and switched to oral medication, and many others who could not (or would not) be controlled through dietary measures alone also responded favorably to them. Today, these drugs are used successfully by approximately one-third of all diabetic patients. Although it is not clear how, the drugs stimulate the pancreas to create more insulin than it would otherwise. Originally, there were four pills: Dymelor, Orinase, Tolinase and Diabinise, all in the sulfonylurea family of drugs. In the beginning, Diabinise caused problems of water and salt retention, but this is not the case with a second generation of sulfonylurea compounds introduced in this country five years ago: glipizide and glyburide. In addition, these newer pills may be given in much smaller doses—one-hundreth of the dose of the first-generation pills. This is a great benefit, because the lower dose reduces the possible side effect of abnormal heart rhythm.

I have concerned myself chiefly with drugs and their use in this chapter, but there are a great many more questions on the patient's mind: How do I keep control of my diabetes? What can I eat and drink? If I have diabetes, will my children have it too? How do I avoid complications? What if my child already has diabetes? What about exercise? Why do different doctors give me different instructions? All these questions and many others will be answered in the following chapters. Let's begin with the first one: control.

3
KEEPING CONTROL

KEEPING CONTROL OF diabetes requires vigilance in regard to blood-sugar readings. What blood-sugar readings signify good control of diabetes? There are many variables to be considered. Not only must patients be weighed and their blood sugar measured individually by their physician, but conditions of the moment must be considered: does the patient have a fever? Is she taking medication? Is he under unusual tension? These are some of the questions that must be asked. Only the patient's doctor knows the precise range of his or her readings. In general, however, the aim for most patients should be a premeal blood sugar of 60–100 milligrams per deciliter, a reading that would be expected to rise to 140–180 milligrams per deciliter one hour after a meal, and fall back to 120–150 two hours after a meal. In response to treatments for the newly diagnosed diabetic, these readings may be forthcoming almost immediately, but it is not uncommon for adjustments to continue over a four-month period before control is achieved.

When this control is realized, how can it be maintained? The answer is a carefully tailored regimen of diet, exercise and insulin (or oral diabetes medication) that also includes regular testing to keep track of blood-glucose levels. Testing is a vital part of this program, for without it neither doctor nor patient can know when adjustments in regimen, especially in regard to insulin, are required. But many newly diagnosed diabetics find the need for such adjustments both puzzling and annoying.

"Once weeks are spent trying to find the right program for control of my diabetes," they say, "why should it have to be changed? Why can't I get one schedule and stick with it, to keep everything easy to remember and follow?"

The answer is purely physical: the body changes. And it changes even if we eat precisely the same foods, perform precisely the same amount of exercise, live in precisely the same environment. Proof of this can be seen in the fact that even under the strict conditions followed by half the patients in the recent DCCT study, their blood-glucose levels fluctuated markedly. As surely and simply as our appetites vary and our taste preferences change from week to week or day to day or even hour to hour, so too do many physical conditions such as the level of glucose in our blood.

When the body is working properly, the islets in the pancreas adjust to these changes in glucose, supplying insulin or shutting it off as sugar in the blood rises or falls. Within reason, the diabetic's aim should be to try to match the body's normal functioning. This does *not* mean striving for "perfect" sugar readings. Such a goal is unreasonable. Occasional unexplained high blood sugars are just part of having diabetes. What patients should work for is to have *most* of their glucose readings within the range agreed upon by their doctor. That will be possible only with regular testing of blood-glucose levels.

Up until twelve years ago, the only practical method for self-testing was via the urine, a method that continues to be widely used today. With urine testing, a chemically impregnated strip is dipped into a sample of urine. The resulting color change of the strip is then compared with a chart that indicates the glucose level. It is a relatively simple test, but it is not without serious shortcomings.

To begin with, a test of the urine cannot determine how high or low the blood-glucose level is *at the moment*. The period required for the kidneys to manufacture urine means that the product being examined on that coated strip is advising the patient what his or her blood glucose level was *several hours previously*. It may well be much higher or lower at the moment of testing. Thus, any steps taken to correct the sugar level could be dangerously out of date.

I vividly recall the day the wife of a forty-year-old newly diagnosed diabetic came to me very near to tears. "Our doctor told me how important it is for my husband to test his urine," she said nervously. "The doctor wants the tests done three times a day and a record kept. But my husband has stopped doing it. Another salesman where he works says the tests aren't accurate, so why bother? So now my husband gets irritated if I keep after him to follow the doctor's orders, but then the doctor criticizes me when my husband doesn't do it. I'm at my wits' end."

The other salesman, it turned out, was also a diabetic and had been told by his doctor that urine tests were virtually worthless in the control of diabetes. Even worse, that doctor told his patient that control of diabetes was not really important; that so long as the patient's regime was sufficient to avoid coma, that was enough.

Shocking? Actually the doctor was far from alone in this opinion. He was expressing one side of an argument that divided the medical community for three-quarters of a century. In question were the complications that are too often the result of long-term diabetes: kidney disease, blindness, nerve and blood-vessel damage, crippling leg pain, gangrene, even leg amputations. Are these complications caused by some unknown aspect of the disease, or are they caused by too much sugar in the blood for a prolonged period? And if the latter is the case, can diabetics avoid these complications by keeping their sugar levels near normal?

Many doctors insisted the complications were due to that unknown aspect of diabetes, and that nothing could be done to prevent the complications. But many other doctors, including myself, believed that with proper control, diabetics could live a long and active life with no more complications than nondiabetics. Since there was no sufficiently persuasive research on the subject, those who believed in control generally did so because of results they had seen in their own practice or in that of physicians who had come before them. Based on this kind of evidence, many of us were firmly convinced that control was the key to a normal future for the diabetic. But how was this control to be achieved?

The answer came in the early 1980s with the discovery that a person's blood-sugar level could be measured by looking at the percentage of red blood cells that are attached to sugar molecules. (Normally, a person's blood contains about 5 or 6 percent of these cells, with very little change; but in diabetics, the figures can easily fluctuate from 7 to 13 percent or even higher.) What this discovery led to was a portable, book-sized machine that can, with the prick of a finger, read a patient's blood-glucose level! Finally, timely blood self-testing had arrived for the diabetic, and it was both simple and accurate.

Not only did this development make possible control by way of accurate self-testing; it also made possible a research project to determine whether such control would, as many of us believed, have a positive effect on a diabetic's future in terms of complications. So long as self-testing had been limited to unreliable urine strips (and blood testing could only be handled by a hospital or doctor's office), research on a sufficiently large scale had been virtually impossible. Now, at last, such a program could be carried out.

Financed by the National Institute of Diabetes and Digestive and Kidney Diseases, a ten-year $160 million research project got underway in 1983. "It was," says the Institute's director, Dr. Phillip Gorden, "the largest and most important study undertaken in the history of diabetes."

Conducted at twenty-nine centers in the United States and Canada, the project (DCCT) recruited 1,441 people, all with Type 1 diabetes, some with no signs of complications from the disease, others with hints that complications were beginning. The average age of the diabetic was twenty-seven, and half of those chosen were women. Each of the patients was randomly assigned to one of two groups, groups that were quite different in the way they approached the concept of control.

The first group handled the diabetes in almost the only manner that had been practical prior to the availability of blood-glucose machines: they followed an unchanging schedule in terms of diet, exercise and insulin injections (once or twice per day), testing their blood sugar only once "as a daily benchmark and to be certain it was not at a dangerous level." But those in the second group tested their blood sugar four or five times per day, adjusting their insulin dosage "as needed." This meant that in an effort to keep their blood-sugar level as close to normal as possible, they took anywhere from three to five insulin injections daily. The idea was not to take in *more* insulin, but to deliver it in a manner that more closely imitated the body's normal release of the hormone by adjusting the insulin dose (and sometimes diet or exercise) when sugars were too high or too low.

The second group of patients worked very closely—much more so than the first group—with their doctors, nurses and dieticians, who phoned them one or more times every week. This consultation was especially important in terms of interpreting the blood-glucose readings, thereby determining the amount of insulin needed. The aim was *not* to respond to a single high or low reading, but rather to respond to *patterns*—readings taken over an extended period of time and interpreted by the doctors and nurses.

Over the life of the research, on an average, the tight control group kept blood sugar at 7.2 percent, or 155 milligrams per deciliter. These figures are startling when compared with those for the more loosely controlled group: 8.9 percent, or 231 milligrams per deciliter. This shows a dramatic difference.

The test was scheduled to continue for a full ten years, but the results were so remarkable that the project was halted a year early to allow all diabetics to benefit from the findings. And what were they? The second group—the group that carefully monitored and sought to control blood sugar—reduced the onset of serious complications by an average of 50 to 60 percent! Some were even able to *reverse* mild kidney disease.

"The discovery of insulin was an absolute miracle," says Dr. Gorden, "and the results of the study are in the ballpark of comparison."

Although the study involved only Type 1 diabetes, there is no doubt that the results are applicable to Type II diabetics, especially those using insulin. "It's the casual approach of many Type II diabetics that puts them in jeopardy," says Dr. James Gavin II, current president of the American Diabetes Association. "The DCCT shows clearly that it's important for *all* people with diabetes to bring their blood sugar close to normal."

Once and for all, this research has proven conclusively that diabetics need not fear the future, need not have their psyches scarred by shocking stories of inescapable complications. The DCCT study proves that, with proper control, those potentially devastating complications can be prevented, or, at the very least, postponed indefinitely. Was it very difficult for the patients to follow this tight control schedule? Listen to the answer from Tracy Sankstone, a twenty-seven-year-old diabetic who was the first person selected for the research in 1983. "Doing four blood tests and four or more shots was tough in the beginning," he says, "but we got into it very quickly. And I'm used to it now. I feel great. I don't have any complications, and I don't want to get them."

Think about what all this means to newly diagnosed diabetics! Think of how their future lives have been improved over just the past ten years: no more dependency on unreliable urine testing or being forced to trek to the hospital or doctor's office whenever there was a need for blood testing. And no more debates between doctors about whether control of diabetes can truly mean the kind of complications-free future many of us were promising even before the research had been undertaken.

"It is extraordinarily exciting," says Dr. David M. Nathan, an associate professor at Harvard Medical School and the principal investigator of the DCCT project. "This kind of thing comes along only once in a lifetime."

Now, more than ever, there is no reason why anyone, patient or relative, should suffer from diabetic neurosis.

A Warning

Except for use in testing for ketones (discussed a bit later), I cannot recommend the use of urine strips in the control of diabetes. I stress this point here for three reasons:

1. Some recently published materials have recommended the use of these strips for those who

do not feel able to exercise "strict control" over their diabetes.
2. The strips remain the blood-sugar measurement choice for many diabetics because there is no large initial cash outlay (no machine).
3. The strips are preferred by many men because they can be carried in the pocket and are simple to use in any men's room.

Regardless of these factors, I strongly urge all diabetics to change to blood-testing machines as used in the DCCT study. The danger with urine strips goes beyond the fact that they are delivering "yesterday's news" which the diabetic tends to treat as current information. Additional shortcomings include the fact that the change of color produced by the urine is sometimes difficult to "read," and this problem may be compounded by medication such as Vitamin C, which can distort results. But perhaps the most misleading factor of all is urine *volume*. If the patient has recently drunk a large amount of water, the same amount of sugar can have a lower concentration than in a lesser volume of urine.

No wonder use of these urine strips often leads to diabetic neurosis. Even though the patient carries out the test by following instructions to the letter, his or her "readings" may be hopelessly confusing or far away from the results desired by both patient and doctor. When this happens, patients often feel they are disappointing their families, their doctors and, worst of all, themselves. They tend to assume responsibility for the failure—which leads to frustration, guilt, anxiety and a very unhappy day-to-day existence.

Ed, a thirty-four-year-old plumber who monitored

his blood sugar via urine strips, nervously told me this story on his first visit to my office. "My diabetes has been very unpredictable, with wild swings from heavy sugar to insulin reactions. Not long ago, while I had a sore throat, very heavy sugar began to appear in my urine. Despite the fact that I ate very little, the tests continued to show sugar. Finally, I had to go to the hospital. I was very ill and had to be given large amounts of insulin and fluid in the vein. I don't want that to happen again."

Ed's "wild swings" were at the root of his trouble, and these grew out of the fact that he was using urine strips to test for blood sugar. Upon finding high glucose, according to the strips, he became highly agitated, berated himself for eating the wrong foods and began restricting his diet so severely that he soon suffered hypoglycemia. In other words, he went from one extreme to another, and the result was hospitalization.

Despite the cost, which averages about seventy-five dollars, diabetics should purchase a blood-glucose meter. Health insurance may cover the expense, but even if it does not, the testing device will pay for itself many times over.

ADDITIONAL TESTS

As an important part of control, we must talk about two other tests: those for ketones and glycosylated hemoglobin.

Ketones

In adhering to the diabetic regimen, it is important that the patient avoid dangerously low blood sugars, for this leads to the formation of ketones, the chemical by-product of the body's burning fat instead of sugar for energy, and one of the earliest signs of potential diabetic complications. Although patients are generally aware of any low blood sugars that occur during waking hours, the same cannot be said of the period during sleep. It is for this reason that I recommend urine testing (strips) for my patients using insulin. Type 1 diabetics should do these tests twice each week, just after rising. If ketones turn up regularly in their urine, a reduction in insulin dosage near bedtime is indicated. Adult-onset diabetics should do such testing at least during periods of illness, when the results of their normal regimen may be distorted.

Glycosylated Hemoglobin

The use of today's self-testing blood-glucose machines four times per day provides far more knowledge than patients and doctors had ten years ago. But still more information is needed by the doctor. Bear in mind that prior to the time a patient developed diabetes, his or her pancreas was "testing" every minute of the day to determine insulin needs. Although artificial methods cannot match this, we can help, with a special test that provides a relatively clear picture of how successful control has been during the past few weeks. This is the glycosylated-hemoglobin test.

Red blood cells have a life span of 120 days, and, depending on the amount of glucose in the blood, these cells become what might be called "sugar-coated"—that is, glycosylated. If a patient has been able to keep the diabetes under good control during the past few weeks, the sugar-coating would be normal. But if sugar levels consistently have been too high, this will be reflected in the amount of glycosylation.

To take the test, the patient must visit the lab, where a fasting blood sample will be taken. From this, the lab can determine the amount of glycosylation that has been occurring in the blood.

This is an important part of the checks and balances diabetics can use to avoid worrying about whether they may have lost control without realizing it. I recommend a glycosylated test at least twice each year, at times designated by the physician.

Summary

Once the diabetes has been brought under control, it must be regulated through a regimen worked out with the diabetic's doctor that includes

1. Diet
2. Exercise
3. Insulin and/or oral medication
4. Multiple self-tests for blood glucose
5. Regular urine testing for ketones
6. Regular lab testing for glycosylated hemoglobin

To this regimen, let me add three cautions: first, patients should not interpret the fourth step—multiple self-tests for blood glucose—to mean that they will learn to readjust the insulin dosage each time they test for glucose. It is unfortunate that many diabetics draw this erroneous conclusion early on and are unable to shake the idea.

The basic purpose of multiple self-tests each day is to provide a *pattern* that can be compared with days, and even weeks, previous. And it is this comparison that will help patients, along with their doctor and nurse, to adjust and then readjust the insulin dosage. Any attempt to readjust insulin dosage based on a single blood test is fraught with danger. A patient's blood sugar may drop precariously following an injection of extra insulin and, as happens all too frequently in such situations, cause an insulin reaction. Those who might advise a dosage increase based on a single blood test fail to take into consideration the fact that there is a lag of many, many hours before a change of insulin dosage produces any noticeable effect. Thus, the increase in dosage generally fails to reduce blood sugar but often increases the frequency and severity of hypoglycemic episodes—which also serve to increase diabetic neurosis.

A second caution is that the patient should never aim to rid the blood of glucose. As diabetes specialist Dr. Clifford F. Gastineau has pointed out, "The body *must* have a certain amount of carbohydrate and enough insulin to use it. If it does not have *both,* the body starts to burn fat and protein at an excessive rate, and ketone bodies are formed." And the doctor adds: "No major harm seems to be done by brief periods of excess sugar."

A third caution is that, although tight control is vital to proper diabetes care, the regimen should never be interpreted so strictly that it leaves the patient "no room to breathe." Ideally, patients will always test their blood four times per day. But if, on occasion, other important demands intrude, there is nothing wrong with cutting back on testing for a day or two in order to provide that breathing room. True, blood-sugar control will be lessened somewhat during this brief period of relaxation, but in the long run, this will be an acceptable loss if it helps the patient remain positive in terms of attitude toward his or her diabetes and keeping it under control.

4

FOOD AND DRINK
FOR THE DIABETIC

THE ENTIRE SUBJECT of food and drink for the diabetic
is filled with problems defined by the American Medical Association as "nutritional neurosis and food
faddism." No other aspect of life causes the diabetic
and her family so much anxiety, guilt and confusion.

"My cousin is a physician's assistant," a new patient, a very attractive woman in her mid-thirties, told
me, "so the minute I said they'd found sugar in my
urine, my cousin said it was good-bye to happy
eating. No more cake or pie or anything like that.
Just the thought of it depressed me terribly."

"My wife told me I'd have to quit sweets cold,"
said another patient, a large man with a very hearty
appetite. "I haven't had a decent meal since."

Imagine the psychological consequences of such
advice in today's world, where we are bombarded by
constant invitations to eat, drink and consume—on
television, in newspapers and magazines, in the gro-
cery store and restaurant. Aside from any pangs of

personal deprivation, consider what such misinformation means in terms of family togetherness for the diabetic mother who has always drawn great pleasure from preparing special desserts for her family, or for the diabetic father who has always enjoyed going out for an ice cream with his.

"I know I shouldn't eat some of the things I do," says Tom, "but there are lots of subtle pressures most people never even think about." So Tom, like most diabetics, goes on eating so-called "forbidden" food and suffering doubly—first, because of his efforts to restrain himself, and second, because of his guilty conscience each time he fails.

"My son is a teenager," the mother of a diabetic told me. "I can't get him to stick to his diet. It's so confusing, he says he can't even understand it, much less follow it, and I have to agree with him. But it scares me."

Over the years, a special language has grown up around dieting for diabetics. Terms such as *free diets, strict diets* and *diabetic diets* abound, causing misinterpretation by patients, dieticians and physicians alike, and leading to either anger or apathy on the part of many diabetics when they can't follow these diets as "strictly" as they think they should. "I can't take those diabetic diets," new patients often tell me. "They're not fair to me or to my family. They're so structured that they're oppressive. No sweets, all that measuring. It's like having a keeper."

Such diets, which demand that patients alter not only their natural taste preferences but even their lifestyles, are doomed to failure. It is not surprising that 50 to 80 percent of diabetics fail to follow the dietary advice they are given.

These restrictions and prohibitions are equally difficult for the family of the diabetic, who often deny themselves "sweet stuff" for fear of putting temptation in a loved one's way or, just as dangerous psychologically, feel guilty each time they do succumb. "I know it's not fair to the rest of the family," says the mother of an eleven-year-old diabetic daughter, "but if I served any sweet things at the table, it would make me feel terrible for my little girl."

Nor are such problems limited to food. "If I have a drink at home," says the wife of a diabetic, "I try to hide what I'm doing. That makes me feel like an alcoholic—but if I don't hide it, I wonder if my husband is looking at me and feeling deprived." Meanwhile, her husband, the former president of a social club, refuses to go out with his old group of friends. "If I can't take a drink," he explains, "I'll put a damper on everybody else's good time."

So both patients and their families suffer from fear of drinking, embarrassment at not drinking, fear of overeating, fear of undereating, guilt due to "going off my diet," difficulties in staying on it—*and absolutely none of this is necessary.*

The truth is that, with good counseling, a proper understanding of their condition and a reasonable amount of willpower, diabetics can eat and drink in a manner that will not only satisfy their own inner needs, but make their families tend to forget their diabetes—and keep friends and acquaintances totally unaware of it.

The medical evidence is clear: neither sweets nor alcohol are, in themselves, harmful to diabetics. That the forceable removal of these items from the diet can produce severe neurosis in diabetics and their families is ample reason in itself to erase the age-old stigma that adheres to such items. But there are other reasons as well. *The evidence is clear that the removal of such sources of carbohydrate from the diabetic's diet can do him or her physical as well as psychological harm.* It can result in dangerously lowered levels of energy, on the one hand, and increased levels of cholesterol and triglyceride (cholesterol-related fatty acid), on the other.

In view of such evidence, why do so many "authorities" appear to believe otherwise? What is the reason for the layers upon layers of misinformation? Why isn't the truth common knowledge?

The answer lies in the nature and history of diabetes.

Nature and history

Derived from Greek words meaning "passing through honey," the name Diabetes Mellitus refers to the elevated glucose (blood sugar) in a patient's urine. The diabetic patient's surplus glucose passes from the bloodstream through the kidneys into the urine, causing the disease's characteristic symptoms: extreme thirst, hunger, weakness, weight loss and the production of abnormally large amounts of urine.

Let's go back to the last century and try to visualize what a physician thought when faced with the challenge of fighting such a disease. With only a minimal knowledge of the subject and with no blood tests or urinalysis available to verify clinical findings, his diagnostic technique was limited almost entirely to the study of patients' symptoms. Noting a patient's frequent urination, then, he would logically have taken a urine specimen and compared it with one from a normal individual. Perhaps he noted the number of flies attracted to the diabetic's urine, or perhaps he actually tasted the specimen, but for whatever reason, he became aware of the urine's high sugar content.

The conclusion he drew was natural: the source of this excess sugar had to be high-sugar foods consumed by the patient, and so he advised his patients to deny themselves all sweets. Could that physician have been expected to know that the patient's excess blood sugar was due to the shortage of one commodity (insulin), rather than the overabundance of another (sweets)?

"Sweets are poison to the diabetic," reads an ancient medical text. Thus were the seeds of diabetic diet neurosis sown—and their growth would be stimulated by every major medical advance in the field of diabetics.

In 1916, six years before the discovery of insulin, Dr. Frederick M. Allen took several dogs and removed seven-eighths of the pancreas from each. The result: on a normal diet, the dogs went into a diabetic coma and died, but even with only one-eighth of a pancreas they were able to survive and live a normal life span if they were fed a low-calorie diet. This startling principle was then applied with great success to human diabetics.

There are two types of diabetics: the juvenile diabetic, whose pancreas fails to produce any insulin at all; and the adult-onset diabetic (of which there is by far the greater number), whose pancreas produces some—but not enough—insulin. Dr. Allen's low-calorie diet could not save the lives of juvenile, or thin, or normal-weight insulin-deficient diabetics, but for the obese individual whose problem was an over-burdened pancreas producing reduced amounts of insulin, it brought impressive results. In most instances, diabetes control was achieved rapidly, and occasionally the condition even reverted to normal.

The benefits of this diet regimen, as Dr. Allen sought to emphasize throughout his studies, were a result of the low-calorie content and its effect on the overweight condition of the patients. Their diabetic condition improved *because they limited the number of calories they consumed, not because there was a limit on the kinds of food they could enjoy.*

In spite of Dr. Allen's efforts to place emphasis where it belonged, however, his discovery was constantly linked to the ancient theory that sugar in the urine meant sugar in the diet. Because a reduction in carbohydrates almost invariably means a reduction in calories, most medical authorities in America decided that Dr. Allen's experiments had been successful not because they offered a diet low in calories, but because they offered one low in sweets.

Even the great discovery of insulin in 1922 by Banting and Best did not begin to set the record straight. With the lives of insulin-deficient adult and juvenile diabetics now preserved and their primary defect counteracted by way of insulin injections, one would expect that the next logical step in the treatment of diabetes would have been the reassessment and normalization of food and drink consumption.

Instead, the ingrown custom of restricting carbohydrates in diabetic patients persisted—so much so that diabetic children whose insulin deficiency had now been corrected frequently lacked sufficient energy to attend classes because of the low-carbohydrate diets they were prescribed! Worse yet, many of these children, failing to attain normal growth and development, became "diabetic dwarfs."

"Sweets are poison to the diabetic," said the medical history books, and in spite of new discoveries, the authorities refused to believe otherwise.

Not until 1930, almost ten years after the discovery of insulin, was a beginning made in the prescription of larger quantities of carbohydrates for diabetic patients. Dr. Sansum in Santa Barbara, California, pioneered this plan, but the advantages of his diets over the usual noncarbohydrate ones were "discovered" in a most unusual fashion.

It was not uncommon for diabetics who vacationed in California and were cared for by Dr. Sansum to report to their doctors in New York that they had felt much better while vacationing in Santa Barbara, only to revert to feeling fatigued and lethargic after returning home. At first, the New York doctors were inclined to attribute the improved health to the California climate, but ultimately it became clear that the beneficial effects resulted from the additional carbohydrates permitted in Dr. Sansum's diets.

The message was plain: increasing sweets, as long as calories were kept sufficiently low in other ways, not only provided psychological benefits but also reduced lethargy. It was a message soon to be supported by the 1935 high-carbohydrate, low-calorie diet experiments of Dr. Himsworth in England—yet it never filtered down to diabetics and their families. Most medical authorities continued to preach the same old sermon: "Sweets are poison to the diabetic."

"If Western clinicians had been less parochial, we would have appreciated sooner the surprising tolerance of diabetics for dietary carbohydrate when caloric intake is controlled." So says Dr. K. M. West, who reported in 1973 that many Eastern and tropical nations had long known that diabetes could be satisfactorily controlled by diets containing almost twice as much carbohydrate as that in the standard diabetic diets of the West.

The diabetics in one Japanese clinic, for example, obtained 64 percent of their calories from carbohydrates, and in India, clinicians often prescribed diets that contained more than 70 percent carbohydrates. It is worth noting here that a meal of the typical, nondiabetic Asian is low in calories and, in terms of percentage, high in carbohydrates (some 130 to 250 grams)—and that Asians have a very low incidence of diabetes.

Today, evidence of both the physical and psychological benefits of high-carbohydrate, low-calorie diets for diabetics continues to grow. Consider these examples:

- The diabetic patients of Stone and Conner did well on diets in which 65 percent of the calories came from carbohydrates.
- Dr. K. M. West, treating a severe diabetic with malignant hypertension, prescribed a rice diet "out of desperation." Although this increased the patient's dietary carbohydrate by almost 300 percent, no increase in insulin was necessary.
- Much later, Dr. West studied a severely diabetic patient on a standard diabetic diet. After

a suitable period of control in a metabolic ward, the patient's daily carbohydrate intake was doubled (from 180 to 360 grams), which greatly improved the patient's energy level and general sense of well-being yet caused no change in the levels of blood and urine glucose.

- R. L. Weinsier showed that for eighteen diabetic patients, a diet high in carbohydrate (60 percent) did not upset the control of diabetes.
- Some of the most impressive studies are those by J. D. Brunzell and associates (1974). In these experiments, diabetes subjects treated with insulin or oral sulfonylureas all had lower fasting glucose levels while receiving the high-carbohydrate diet than they did when receiving the usual diabetic diet.
- Additional studies have also shown that the high-carbohydrate diets, which are low in fat, significantly decrease the cholesterol and triglyceride levels, which is important for heart and arterial health.

However, even though these medical studies provide conclusive proof that a low-carbohydrate diet is not indicated in the treatment of diabetes—that, in fact, such a diet can be both physically and psychologically injurious—the notion that "sweets are poison" still continues to dominate the thinking of many physicians treating diabetes. Why? Primarily because

- Old superstitions die hard.
- Many physicians see that a restriction of carbohydrate intake results in improvement in the diabetic, but fail to recognize that this is actu-

ally a result of fewer calories rather than fewer sweets.

- It seems common sense to connect sugar in the blood with sugar in the mouth. The correlation between the two appears as irrefutable as the logic which caused a small boy to believe he had caused an East Coast blackout because all the lights went out just as he struck a light pole with his stick.

For these reasons, the false connection between carbohydrates and diabetes, although disproven time and time again, continues to reappear in textbooks and clinics. To this day, the limiting of dietary carbohydrates is the cornerstone of diabetic therapy for many clinicians, dieticians and physicians.

This is not the only restriction to pose mental and physical problems for diabetics and their families, however. There is also the diet regimen itself.

The diets

Many diets prescribed for diabetes not only restrict carbohydrates but also require meticulous calorie counting, very precise measurement of food intake and utilization of complex food exchanges. Since the physician usually emphasizes diet as the keystone of diabetic management, patients and their families naturally jump to the conclusion that whenever they have fluctuations in their glucose readings, errors in calculating food intake, whether accidental or on purpose, are the principal causes.

In truth, however, the human body is a very complex machine that reacts to a vast array of stimuli.

Any attempt to tie changes in blood-sugar levels to fluctuations in food consumption would be as foolish as insisting that we get depressed because we eat corned beef and cabbage.

Contrary to the belief of many, diabetic patients are not likely to gorge themselves with food one day and starve the next, any more than any nondiabetics might. No matter what food idiosyncrasies an individual has, one fact stands out: his or her menu contains almost identical food items, day after day, meal after meal, sometimes to the point of monotony. Most people eat unvarying breakfasts and lunches throughout their lives. Diabetics are as conformist in their eating patterns as anyone else, and the fluctuations in their blood-sugar levels and urine-sugar tests cannot be correlated with hypothetical peaks and valleys in their food intake. When the blood sugar is unduly elevated, the patient's eating habits may be utterly blameless.

There are marked fluctuations in a patient's test results, even in a hospital, yet this is one of the most controlled environments a diabetic patient can encounter. All the food is carefully measured and supervised by a dietician, and even the amount of the patient's physical activity is constant. Certainly the patient should not be held responsible for variations of blood sugar under such controlled conditions, yet variations definitely do occur. How can the patient be blamed?

There are other major areas of confusion. Many years ago more than 150 different diets were being prescribed for diabetics at the Mount Sinai Hospital in Cleveland, Ohio, alone! Most of these diets varied from one another by only a few grams of carbohydrate, protein or fat—prescribed according to the whim of the physician. Imagine the confusion and uncertainty this caused among diabetics and their families as they compared notes. Even today, although the American Diabetes Association has attempted to reduce the number of diets suggested for diabetics, the lack of agreement among experts regarding this subject, as well as many other aspects of dieting, fosters continued uncertainty.

The complexity and confusing aspects of the diets are not their only self-defeating factors. Quite often the diets call for types of food or preparation so different from that required for the rest of the family that they become disruptive. The inclusion of expensive "diabetic foods" can become a financial burden. And, most important, too often doctors and dieticians fail to tailor a diet to fit the bodily requirements and life-style of the patient. Men who require 2500 or more calories per day for good health, for example, are given diets containing only 1800 calories. Such errors are made for thin men as well as for heavy women and children. Why?

First, many physicians fail to take into account the relationship between calorie requirements and such factors as body size and amount of normal daily exercise.

Second, doctors and dieticians, as well as patients themselves, may overlook the special caloric needs of underweight diabetics.

Third, and of striking importance, many patients are sent home from the hospital on a prescription—such as an eighteen-hundred-calorie ADA diet—that satisfied them perfectly while they were inactive in the hospital, but that will be dangerously deficient to support daily activities at home.

Fourth, the increased bulk of the diabetic diet may actually offer a volume of food equal to that to which the patient had been accustomed on a normal diet. For this reason, most diabetics are initially satisfied with diets offering only 70 to 80 percent of their actual caloric requirement. But the key word here is *initially*. Dissatisfaction soon sets in as the patient is faced with mounting hunger and fatigue.

Small wonder that although all diabetics may claim to be "on a diet," a giant percentage of them do not follow their prescribed diets. The statistical evidence is clear:

- A National Health Survey in Holland showed that 25 percent of the diabetics, although admitting they had received a diet from their physician, did not follow it, while another 22 percent insisted they had never been given a diet at all.
- Among a representative group of American diabetics, 47 percent failed to follow any prescribed diet.
- Dr. Harvey Knowles and his colleagues summarized seven studies of juvenile diabetics which showed that 22 to 89 percent failed to follow their diets.
- In a British study (Tunbridge), the variances in consumption of 70 percent of the prescribed amounts of food for diabetics was more than 10 percent.
- Studies of the University Group Diabetes Program showed that although significant weight

reduction was achieved among the subgroups during the first few days and weeks, old habits soon took over, and as the months passed, adiposity (being overweight) returned.

In many ways, the best of the so-called diabetes diets is the old Exchange Diet, developed conjointly by the American Diabetes Association (ADA), the American Diabetic Association and the United States Public Health Service. It contains all the essential food ingredients—carbohydrates as well as proteins, fats, fruits, vegetables and dairy. The regimen is called an Exchange Diet because it offers a long list of food items that based on their calorie count and protein, carbohydrate and fat content, are interchangeable, thus providing considerable variety.

Even with this diet, however, the complications are such that patients often find it oppressive. Many hours are consumed in attempting to teach patients the mechanics of the exchange system and elements such as "carbohydrate counting." In addition, although the ADA, having "discovered" that carbohydrate in the diet has no meaningful relationship to diabetes, has liberalized its diets over the past fifteen years, it continues to be biased against carbohydrates and toward fats. Moreover, until 1993, the ADA fell prey to the old sweets-are-poison falsehood and advised omission of a long list of "concentrated sugars" such as candy, molasses, honey, jam, jelly, marmalade, syrup, pie, cake, cookies, pastries, table sugar, condensed milk, soft drinks and candy-coated gum—none of which need be restricted, provided their caloric value is taken into account.

Fortunately, a 1993 study by the University of

Minnesota was sufficient to convince the ADA (as many of us were convinced by studies made in the 1970s) that eating table sugar and other products in its "concentrated sugars" list does not increase blood glucose in diabetics any more than eating other starches does, so long as calories are counted. In other words, you can eat a piece of cake in place of a potato if you choose, without suffering ill effects.

It is interesting to note that many of the participants in the University of Minnesota study were so brainwashed by the old sugar-is-poison refrain that they found it extremely difficult to do what they were told. "People in the study were reluctant at first to eat sugar—to put it on their cereal or to eat a brownie, with its thick frosting," says Dr. John P. Bantle, associate professor of medicine at the University of Minnesota. "These were people who had been told to avoid sugar. It was not in their diet. But in the interest of science, they managed to choke down that brownie."

Dr. Bantle's study showed that the belief about sugar being dangerous stemmed from a false assumption, which was that sugars are digested and absorbed rapidly because of their simple structure while starches were digested and absorbed slowly because of their complex nature. Knowing that the more quickly food is digested and absorbed, the more quickly blood glucose levels rise, many physicians assumed that sugars would cause blood glucose to rise faster than would starches. Not true. Whether simple or complex, the structure of the carbohydrate does not matter.

It should be noted that almost every diabetes book available continues to support this fallacy about the danger of simple carbohydrates. But at least the correct information is being used to revise the ADA diets, which should eventually trickle down to millions of sugar-starved diabetics.

The following is what I believe to be the best step-by-step approach to the subject of food and drink.

The Best Approach

PATIENT'S WEIGHT

Before a diet can be prescribed, it is essential to know whether the patient is underweight, overweight or of normal weight. How is this determination to be made? It is unwise to use the familiar insurance tables for height and weight, since the medical profession has determined that these tables are inaccurate. Insurance companies developed these tables simply by tabulating the weights of their applicants and then drawing an average, and since a cross-section of the American population is overweight, the tables are bound to reflect this obesity. If one must use such a table, then the "ideal weight" is the most satisfactory choice. These weights represent a group of insured who "outlived" their life expectancies (further indication that obesity reduces one's life).

A better and simpler method, however, is simple observation and judgment by the diabetic and his or her family. Surprisingly, any group of lay persons will concur as to whether a given individual is underweight, overweight or normal. I have found a very substantial unanimity, for example, among nurses or medical students as to what a patient's weight should be.

At first glance, this method may appear to be too

imprecise and unscientific; however, there is one important factor that makes it highly recommended: it works.

IF THE PATIENT IS UNDERWEIGHT

The underweight diabetic, like any other undernourished person, requires not only sufficient food for daily physical activities but additional calories for gaining weight and strength.

Often, the underweight diabetic will regain her weight without an increase in caloric consumption as her diabetes is brought under control by the administration of insulin or oral medication. If this is not the case, however, I prefer to augment the current diet (provided it is nutritionally sound) by additional calories rather than by substituting a totally new diet. At first, I simply increase food portions at mealtime and between meals, and if this is not sufficiently productive, I increase the fat content of the diet.

Once the patient has reached normal weight, she should follow the advice that follows for those without weight problems.

IF THE PATIENT IS OVERWEIGHT

This category includes the vast majority of diabetics. Weight reduction is the prime treatment for their diabetes, and they must adhere strictly to a low-calorie diet—but only until they have achieved their normal weight. The low-calorie diet should be just as well-balanced nutritionally as any diet, diabetic or not, and it is important to remember that any diet of less than eight hundred calories is unlikely to be able to provide enough essential nutrients to maintain the body over a long period of time without destroying important muscle and other tissue.

I have employed an unlimited-meat diet with very good success for many years. By consuming lean meat, fish, chicken and skim milk, a patient will automatically get sufficient protein while at the same time restricting animal fat and cholesterol in his system (see the diet on page 75). Such a diet, while providing all the normal food constituents, also helps the patient establish proper eating habits, to be continued after he has attained normal weight and is able to follow a maintenance diet.

For the overweight diabetic who regularly follows such a diet, the results are frequently dramatic—in many instances going so far as to reverse the entire diabetic process for an indefinite period. To all intents and purposes, the patient functions as a normal individual.

Once proper weight has been attained, the patient should follow the directions that follow for the normal-weight diabetic.

IF THE PATIENT'S WEIGHT IS NORMAL

The diabetic's diet, like that of any individual, should be well balanced nutritionally and contain adequate amounts of protein, carbohydrates, fats, fruits, vegetables and minerals. Since, as we discussed earlier, the type of food has no bearing on diabetic control, no restrictions of this sort are necessary. But how many calories per day should the normal-weight diabetic consume?

Various formulas have been proposed for predicting the caloric requirements of individuals. Many physicians have been indoctrinated to speak of food prescribed to diabetics in terms of "grams per kilogram of body weight," but Dr. F. F. Davidoff points out the shortcomings of this method: "It's so far removed [from everyday life] that I've never learned the system myself. I've tried, but it just boggled my mind. And I don't think I should try to foist anything on patients that is so hard for me, particularly when cutting it that fine doesn't make much difference. It is my impression that only a minority of medical people still teach students to calculate food to the nearest few grams."

The system of calculating calories strictly on weight has other fallacies as well: for one thing, a person requires progressively fewer calories with increasing age; for another, the patient's type of employment makes a difference. An athlete or manual laborer requires more food than a bookkeeper.

In the final analysis, the best guide to the proper caloric level of a diet is the indicator on the scale. From the very beginning, the patient should develop the habit of daily weigh-ins, and an increase or decrease in weight should dictate a compensatory increase or decrease in calories.

The normal-weight patient, therefore, should simply make sure the diet being followed is well balanced nutritionally and keep a close eye on the scale. Anything more complicated than that is superfluous.

ADDITIONAL MEALS FOR THE DIABETIC

Food is also very important in counteracting the hypoglycemic effect of insulin and oral diabetes drugs. No matter which medication is used, a period of several hours without food may lower the blood sugar precariously; thus it is strongly recommended that the patient eat at regular intervals between meals.

Patients on regular insulin should snack two and one-half hours after the insulin injection, and those on intermediate insulins—NPH, Lente, and 70/80—should snack seven hours afterward. With oral drugs, the patient should simply take something between meals and at bedtime.

If prolonged effect is needed, the mid-meal snack should consist primarily of protein and/or fat: carbohydrates simply do not last long enough.

DIABETIC FOODS

One of the ongoing dietary misconceptions is that regarding so-called "diabetic foods." This assumes that carbohydrates are harmful, and results in many ingenious attempts to reduce the carbohydrate content of foods and sell them to the diabetic at excessive prices.

Aside from water-packed fruits, which simply eliminate sugar solutions and syrup, these foods basically substitute a form of sugar that breaks down more slowly for those foods that produce glucose—the so-called "harmful" sugar. These substitute sugars seldom alter the caloric content of the diet, but obese diabetic patients draw the erroneous conclusion that as long as they use them, they are on the right track. Not so.

Also, many patients are convinced that because these ersatz foods cost more, they must be more valuable. Again, not so. They are simply overpriced and, as far as the diabetic is concerned, useless.

The American Diabetes Association itself advises against the use of "diabetic foods" in its Exchange Diets, recommending instead that the diabetic select food from the same sources used by other members of the family. I heartily concur.

ALCOHOL

In almost every diet prescribed for diabetic patients there appears the phrase, "No alcoholic drinks," with no further explanation given. Patient and physician alike can only infer from this that alcohol somehow raises the blood sugar and affects diabetes adversely—but this is not true.

The fact is that the fate of alcohol in the human body is still something of a mystery. Its end products are carbon dioxide and water, *not* sugar. It is true that some alcoholic beverages, such as beer and wine, contain sugar-producing substances, but even they have no greater ill-effects on diabetes than other carbohydrates, which have been shown to be innocuous.

Although the intake of alcohol has been reported to cause nausea and dizziness in some people, it is only fair to point out that two recent studies have indicated that modest consumption of alcohol—one or two drinks per day—appears to have a beneficial effect in terms of the heart. Perhaps more important here is the fact that even if told to stop drinking entirely, most diabetics do not. They simply sneak a drink here and there, feeling guilty all the while, convinced that they are doing themselves untold harm even while they are taking "a quick one."

It is my custom to permit alcoholic beverages in moderation to all diabetics on a normal caloric diet. If the occasion calls for a little social drinking, then there's no reason not to enjoy yourself!

I would add only two cautions: Alcoholic beverages aren't "free"—the calories do count. And keep in mind that even a single drink has a tendency to lower one's resistence to temptation. If the use of alcohol leads to more than a drink or two per day or to the breakdown of other forms of diabetic control, then the use of alcohol should be discontinued entirely.

The Goodman "Meat Unlimited" Weight-Loss Diet

Note: Avoid fatty, fried, breaded foods as well as food in barbecue sauce or cream. Avoid also stews, casserole dishes and thickened gravy.

BREAKFAST

Fruit (*see Fresh Fruit List for portion and choice*)
1 egg, hard-boiled, poached, scrambled, soft-boiled, prepare without butter
Toast, without crusts—1 piece or ½ bagel
Tea or coffee without cream or sugar
Skim milk—8 ounces

LUNCH

Lean meat, poultry or fish (*see Meat or Fish List*)
1 vegetable (*Vegetable List One or Two*) 1 cup of fat-free vegetable soup or chicken soup may be substituted for 1 vegetable (*Vegetable List Two*)
1 salad (*Vegetable List One*)
Fruit—1 portion (*see Fresh Fruit List*)

DINNER

Lean meat, poultry or fish (*see Meat or Fish List*)
1 vegetable (*see Vegetable List One or Two*) 1 cup of fat-free vegetable soup or chicken soup may be substituted for 1 vegetable (*Vegetable List Two*)

1 salad (*Vegetable List One*)
Fruit—1 portion (*see Fresh Fruit List*)
Tea or coffee without cream or sugar.

EVENING SNACK
Skim milk or low-fat buttermilk—8 ounces.

Spices, vinegar and low-calorie salad dressing may be
used as desired. Vegetables are to be cooked in water or
low-sodium bouillon; no sauce or butter is to be added.

VEGETABLE LIST ONE
(1 measuring cup)

Artichoke, fresh
Asparagus
* Beet greens
* Broccoli
Brussels sprouts
Cabbage
* Carrot sticks, raw
Cauliflower
Celery

* Chicory or endive
Cucumbers
* Dandelions
Eggplant
* Escarole
Green Onions
* Kale
* Leeks
Lettuce

VEGETABLE LIST TWO
(½ measuring cup)

Beets
* Carrots

* Pumpkin
Rutabaga

---

*These vegetables contain large amounts of vitamin A. Use
one every day.

Kohlrabi
Onions
Peas, small

* Squash, winter
Turnips

FRESH FRUIT LIST
(Two portions daily)

Apple, small—1
Apricot, medium—2
Berries—1 cup
† Cantaloupe or water-
melon—1 cup
Cherries—1 cup
† Grapefruit, small—½
Grapes—15
† Lemon, lime, large—1

† Orange, small—1
Peach, medium—1
Pear, small—1
Pineapple—1 slice
Plum, medium—2
Prunes—3
† Tangerine, large—1

MEAT LIST
(Any amount, boiled, broiled or roasted)

Hint: Trim all fat from meat; remove skin from
duck, chicken, turkey

Beef
Brain
Chicken
Kidney

Lamb
Liver
Turkey
Veal

---

†These fruits contain large amounts of vitamin C. Use one
every day.

FISH LIST
(Any amount, but no other kinds)

Carp

Cod

Crabmeat

Flounder

Haddock

Halibut

Lobster

Oysters

Perch

Pike

Scallops

Shrimp

Smelt

Trout

Whitefish

FREE
(The following foods may be eaten anytime, in any amount)

Lean meat

Fish

Poultry

Vegetables List One

Dill or sour pickles

Coffee

Tea

Clear bouillon

Diet soft drinks

Note: Seasonings can be very helpful in making food taste better, but beware of sodium. Read labels, and choose both foods and seasonings low in sodium.

For hints on feeding children, see Chapter Seven.

5

MARRIAGE AND CHILDREN

ONE NEED NOT have a degree in psychiatry in order
to be familiar with the painful emotional problems
encountered by many young people as they mature,
fall in love and begin to look ahead toward the possibility of marriage and creating their own families.
The passions and confusions experienced by Romeo
and Juliet are just as real today as they were when
Shakespeare wrote about them.

Now add to this highly emotional period something such as diabetes. To those in their late teens or
early twenties, the announcement, almost always totally unexpected, that they are negatively different—
that they must spend the rest of their lives dependent
on injections and special regimentation—can be dangerously traumatic unless it is accompanied by an
honest picture of what diabetes is really like and the
marvelous strides that have been made in the field in
recent years.

All too often, however, the very opposite occurs.
The announcement of diabetes is accompanied by
only a minimum of information, or, worse, by dis-

torted data and advice that, however well intentioned, are totally out of date. Imagine what this means to those young adults:

"I was seventeen when they discovered I had diabetes," says Linda, a very bright, attractive young woman. "I had already planned my life. I was going to attend a midwestern university, work as a reporter, travel a lot and then, I hoped, marry and have children." But the doctor's pronouncement, cold and impersonal, threw ice water on Linda's plans. "I didn't think any man would want to marry someone with an incurable disease, and that's how I began to look at my illness—not as something that could be controlled, but as an incurable disease. I decided I would devote my life to a career only."

Another young woman, a secretary in an insurance office, found that the announcement of her diagnosis made her feel like a criminal. "The way the whole thing was described, with needles and all that, made me picture myself like a drug addict. I felt guilty and dirty, and I didn't want anybody to find out about it. I knew I couldn't get married. I cried a lot, and I thought about suicide."

Even if the young diabetic is willing to keep an open mind about the possibility of marriage, his or her parents may not be. Concerned not only for their child's physical well-being but also for the emotional damage they foresee as a result of diabetes, many parents become overprotective.

"My mom tried to turn me off of every girl I dated," says a young man whose diabetes was diagnosed only five days before his eighteenth birthday. "She was so afraid the girls would leave me flat when they found out about my being a diabetic that she tried to keep me from getting serious with anyone.''

His mother admits that she interfered, but explains the situation differently. ''It wasn't just that the disease might be repugnant to the girls he liked. I worried that they wouldn't be willing to give my son the treatment he needed, to watch over him the way I was doing.''

For most healthy-minded young people, the prospect of marriage is accompanied by the thought of raising one's own family. How does the advent of diabetes affect such considerations?

''I know my boyfriend would want children,'' said a young schoolteacher who, only recently diagnosed as a diabetic, was now reluctant to accept a marriage proposal. ''I wouldn't want to fail him as a wife, and I've heard it's almost impossible for diabetic women to become pregnant. Would it be fair for me to marry him?''

And while this young teacher worried that she might not be able to become pregnant, her mother's fears were focused in precisely the opposite direction—on the complications that might ensue if her daughter did become pregnant. ''A friend of mine had an aunt who was diabetic,'' the mother told me, ''and she almost died during her pregnancy. There were all sorts of complications. And then the baby was oversized and they had to take it by Cesarean.''

Fears such as these do not stem solely from old wives' tales. Many physicians themselves pass on similarly frightening information to their patients, or even to other doctors. ''Women with severe diabetes should be strongly advised to avoid pregnancy,'' Dr. Paul Beck told the Eighth Congress of the International Diabetes Federation meeting in Brussels in 1973. Dr. Beck, an associate professor of medicine at the University of Colorado, stressed not only the possible complications of pregnancy but also warned against "adding to the genetic pool of diabetics" (passing on diabetes to one's offspring).

Of all the myths surrounding marriage and childbearing for diabetics, there is probably none more well entrenched than the "fact" that the disease is hereditary. "It's in our genes," a twenty-four-year-old bride told me tearfully. "My husband has it, and now we've found out my mother's sister had it too. We don't dare have children. And it's tearing our marriage apart."

In some cases, the marriage never takes place. Upon finding out his daughter had diabetes, a minister insisted that she break off her engagement. "My wife and I feel guilty enough as it is," he explained. "We know diabetes is hereditary, so we are responsible for our daughter's having it. That's terrible enough. We certainly don't want her doing the same thing to more kids. Marriage and children are out of the question."

One of the most depressing examples of misinformation is contained in the following statement made to a twenty-one-year-old college student, mentioned earlier in Chapter One. A gynecologist, upon learning about the student's diabetes in the course of taking a history for a routine examination, immediately sat her down and volunteered this advice: "Since you have diabetes, you must carefully weigh the problems of marriage. You probably can't conceive. And if you do, there are all the dangers associated with pregnancy in diabetics—acidosis, hypertension, hydramnios and so on. If you should manage to over-come all these hazards, the baby probably will not live. If it does, it will be afflicted with congenital deformities.''

Imagine that young woman's reaction to such an announcement. Before this, she had been psychologi-cally well adjusted to her diabetes, but now she was frightened. A friend suggested that she seek another opinion, so she came to me. I recall vividly how, on her first visit to my office, she sank into a chair, repeated what the gynecologist had told her and then looked me directly in the eye.

''Was he right, Dr. Goodman? Tell me the truth. I'm all worn out just thinking about it. I'm going out with a young man, and we're talking about marriage. What about having children?''

As is so often the case, my job with this young woman was not simply to tell her the truth. In order to reopen the future she deserved, I had to spend many hours over many weeks and months undoing the psychic trauma inflicted on her by her gynecolo-gist. To effect a ''cure'' of her diabetic neurosis, it was not enough to give her the facts; I first had to explain the background that could have led her gyne-cologist to frighten her as he did.

The background

All the authentic data show that diabetic females have normal fertility and can become pregnant as readily as nondiabetics. Why, then, would any doctor suggest the opposite? Was there a time when juvenile diabetics had difficulty conceiving?

The answer is, sadly, that there was a time when

juvenile diabetic patients had difficulty doing anything at all. Before the discovery of insulin, pregnancy was almost unheard-of in diabetic patients, simply because they did not live long enough to conceive. The entire life span of the young adult with diabetes was usually limited to a few weeks or, at most, a few months. The question was not how to help the young diabetic conceive, but how to help her live.

With the miraculous discovery of insulin by Banting and Best, the survival rate of young adults immediately began to increase. Long before physicians had achieved a full understanding of the best care for insulin-injecting patients, pregnancy became commonplace among young diabetic women. But there were major problems.

It took time to gain an in-depth understanding of the best use of this new insulin, and even more time to spread this information to the nation's thousands of hospitals and millions of doctors and diabetic patients. While this process of learning and dissemination took place, pregnant diabetics suffered frequently from episodes of ketoacidosis—an extreme type of excess-acid condition that can lead to air-hunger and coma—and hypoglycemia. The mother's life was in constant jeopardy, to such a dramatic extent that simply surviving a pregnancy was hailed as a truly outstanding achievement.

It is this history, stemming from the immediately postinsulin discovery period, then, that is the source of so many doctors' rusty stockpiles of misinformation. But times have changed. As diabetes research progressed, so too did the treatment of pregnant diabetic women. Each step forward in the understanding of diet and regimen was a step forward in the treatment of pregnant diabetics, and special research on the subject was conducted as well.

Pregnancy brings with it dramatic changes in many body functions, not the least of which is abnormal glucose readings even in many nondiabetic mothers. The regular injection of insulin amid such physical changes has often produced unexpected results, but through trial and error and some exceptional clinical research, physicians have rapidly improved their techniques for treatment. A relatively normal pregnancy for diabetics began to be predicted with assurance.

Then, however, as the hazards to the diabetic mother decreased dramatically, concern about their offspring grew. It quickly became apparent that many problems were occurring in the fetuses of diabetic mothers. Most striking was the inordinately high mortality rate. Then the records began to show fetuses of excessively large size and weight, and organs—heart, kidneys and so on—that were oversized and prone to congenital deformities. The offspring were generally described as "big, fat and full-faced." Full term, they often weighed more than ten pounds, and even when born prematurely, they weighed seven to nine pounds, due not to excessive accumulation of fluid (edema) but to actual fleshiness and increased length.

There was great danger of prematurity, early respiratory distress, hypoglycemia (usually developing within six hours after birth), congenital malformations, birth trauma and infection. Babies of diabetic mothers were, without question, sick babies.

The prospects for potential diabetic parents were

extraordinarily depressing. Physicians valiantly sought answers to alleviate their anguish, but in the meantime obstetricians reached agreement that the large babies were poor candidates for normal delivery. It seemed wise, they reasoned, to remove the oversized babies by Cesarean section after thirty-six to thirty-eight weeks, thus obviating difficult labor and taking the infant while life was still strong.

This became a generally accepted routine everywhere, even after newer data clearly showed the offspring were still dying postpartum, usually as a result of respiratory failure due to hyaline membrane disease. Eventually, it was discovered that the prematurity associated with early delivery was, in itself, the greatest hazard for all of these children.

Meanwhile, research continued. The first major breakthrough occurred at the Joslin Clinic, when Dr. Priscilla White reported a hormone imbalance in pregnant diabetic women. Dr. White organized a special clinic where she could study this condition, and where, under her personal supervision, diabetic mothers were given special care and treatment, including the administration of estrogen and progesterone.

The result was a surprisingly improved survival rate, but the greatest surprise of all proved to be the true reason for Dr. White's success. Thanks to a subsequent study of pregnant diabetics by Drs. Black and Miller, it became apparent that the improved survival rate was due not to the administration of hormones, but rather to the all-around improvement in diabetic treatment the mothers received: greater consistency in testing techniques, more concern with special diet, careful scheduling of insulin injections, proper courses of exercise, and the like. The secret of normal pregnancy and childbirth for the diabetic mother had proven to be unexpectedly simple: the careful *control* of the mother's diabetes.

Additional documentation was provided by the Hopkins Groups headed by Dr. John E. Tyson. Based on the excellent results they obtained, Dr. Tyson and his colleagues could report in 1974: "In patients with well-controlled diabetes, perinatal mortality is negligible. This prospective study documents that preterm delivery is unnecessary. . . . Vaginal delivery at term is not only possible but preferable when gestational diabetes is well controlled."

In Dr. Tyson's group, this control was such that glucose values were consistently kept below 100 milligrams per deciliter, and this was accomplished entirely by restricting caloric intake, thereby confining weight gain to less than eight ounces per week. Using this regimen, there were no intrauterine or neonatal deaths, with no increase in perinatal mortality or morbidity as the fetus grew and only minimal complications during delivery.

Dr. Tyson and his associates proved that it was not diabetes itself that was the culprit but, rather, extreme, prolonged fluctuations in glucose readings—in other words, poorly controlled diabetes. Freed from the burden of these conditions, none of the babies developed significant complications, congenital malformations or respiratory distress syndromes.

I heartily agree that the fate of the fetus is tied directly to the degree of diabetes control achieved during pregnancy. In my office, I have a photograph album filled with snapshots of the children of diabetic patients. These pictures have been collected over the past thirty-five years, and thanks to the careful control of the mothers' diabetes during pregnancy, all of these snapshots show normal, healthy, vigorous children. The patient-doctor relationship is of extreme importance here. The young mother's peace of mind is a vital part of her care; hence, her physician must be experienced in treating diabetic mothers-to-be and one in whom she has absolute faith.

Today, because of constantly improving techniques, especially in terms of strict control, a pregnant diabetic woman can look forward with great confidence to a normal baby, delivered in perfectly normal fashion at full term. But is it any wonder so few people are aware of this, when Hollywood produces a major movie such as *Steel Magnolias*? In this film, Sally Field played the mother of Julia Roberts, who portrayed a diabetic. Field was constantly concerned about her daughter, who, at the scriptwriter's whim, drifted in and out of insulin shock no matter what control was exercised or what precautions were taken. The mother's concern grew as the daughter married, and turned to near hysteria when Roberts's character became pregnant. Then, according to this totally unrealistic script, despite the greatest effort by Roberts and her husband and doctor, her diabetes went so far out of control during pregnancy that it eventually led to her death!

It is a tragedy that such films and television programs are produced. Poetic license is one thing; deadly distortions, which may lead to diabetic neurosis, are something else again.

Heredity

In 1973, Dr. D. L. Rimoin, distinguished professor of pediatrics and medicine at the University of California at Los Angeles, stated in no uncertain terms that the World Health Organization had been wrong in 1965 when, in order to avoid "adding to the genetic pool of diabetics," it counseled against diabetics' marrying and having children.

I concur wholeheartedly with Dr. Rimoin. My personal clinical experience over many years has convinced me there is no proven hereditary basis for diabetes. Of the diabetic parents I have known who have one or more offspring, not a single child—not one—has developed diabetes. Conversely, a review of the diabetic children I have treated over more than thirty-five years fails to uncover even one parent with diabetes!

Still, as shown earlier, far too many doctors continue to voice the theory that diabetes is hereditary. Only infrequently are diabetic patients encouraged to proceed normally in raising a family. Far more often, they are warned that they will very likely be passing on their handicap to their children. How did such a misconception arise?

The cornerstone of this theory is the frequent occurrence of diabetes in identical twins when one of them has the disease. Elliot Joslin analyzed this incidence in thirty-three sets of identical twins and sixty-three pairs of fraternal twins, Hildegard Berg studied forty-six identical twins and Friedrich Umber worked with nineteen pairs. Although these samples were far too small to provide statistically meaningful data, dangerously broad inferences were drawn from the studies. The medical profession decided—and so advised the public—that diabetes was a hereditary disease and that children inherited diabetes as a recessive characteristic, according to Mendelian law.

This offered frightening prospects for diabetic parents. If diabetes were, as these physicians suggested, an autosomal recessive disease, the risk of diabetes in the offspring of diabetic parents would be considerable. Where only one of the parents was diabetic, one out of four children would be expected to have diabetes, and where both parents were diabetic, three out of four children would be likely to inherit the disease.

Today, as Dr. Rimoin rightly points out, the concept of recessive inheritance can be overturned very easily: by simply noting that, despite the studies that have found diabetes in the children of two diabetic parents, the diabetes occurs too infrequently to support such a theory. The statistically meaningful studies Dr. Rimoin cites for support are far from isolated examples. D. A. Pyke's investigation, reported in 1973, also revealed that the incidence of diabetes in the children of two diabetics is far lower than would be predicted if the disease were inherited as a single recessive gene. The same is true for Joslin's 1959 data and a 1966 English study. Mendelian law simply does not apply to diabetes.

But if the disease is not hereditary, how are we to explain the frequent occurrence in identical twins when one of them has the disease? And what about the recent data indicating that diabetes occurs more frequently in some families than one would expect from chance alone? A Canadian study indicates a three- to fourfold increase in diabetes among the brothers and sisters of diabetics over forty years of age. The study also shows a four- to fivefold increase when onset for the diabetic occurred between the ages of twenty and thirty-nine, and a ten- to fourteenfold increase when onset occurred before the age of twenty. From studies such as these, it appears that brothers and sisters in any family are more likely to have diabetes if any one member has the disease, and that this possibility increases, the younger that member is at the onset.

Without questioning the accuracy of these data, I must point out that they offer no evidence whatsoever about the likelihood of diabetic parents passing on the disease to their offspring. What it does show is that a husband and wife, regardless of whether or not they have diabetes, may have in their gene package some unique combination that tends to produce diabetic children.

What is this unique gene combination? We do not know, and finding out may very well be a long, drawn-out process. Dr. James V. Neel, professor of human genetics at the University of Michigan, has called diabetes "a geneticist's nightmare." There are three basic reasons.

First, due to the great variability in clinical manifestations, there is substantial disagreement as to what actually constitutes a diabetic; that is, where the dividing line should be drawn between the disease and "normality." Dr. Neel, for example, would restrict the interpretation to those cases where there are, or are expected to be, pathological consequences. Other physicians disagree. It is because of such differences that figures showing the incidence of diabetes differ so widely from study to study. Consider the following data:

A diabetic survey in England (1962) reported the frequency of known diabetics as 2 percent in those over seventy years of age, but the U.S. National

Health Survey (1960) reported an incidence of double that (4 percent) for persons in the same age group. Meanwhile, a large-scale survey in Georgia found abnormal glucose tolerance (one "definition" of diabetes) in 7.4 percent of persons over seventy, while another study of a thousand largely ambulatory patients over sixty not known to have diabetes found 8.8 percent with diabetes or "potential diabetes." And in a study conducted by the University of Michigan in Tecumseh, a Michigan community with a population of over seven thousand, it was found that at least 20 percent of the people over forty fulfilled one definition for "potential diabetes," the attainment of hyperglycemic levels one hour after a standard glucose load.

The second problem that makes diabetes a "geneticist's nightmare" is the fact that incidence of the disease becomes more frequent with age, thus making cross-sectional studies in time totally unrepresentative of the true picture. Add to this the tremendous variability in the age of onset within the two major categories—juvenile and adult—and the fact that juvenile diabetes is entirely different from the adult form, and you have considerable confusion.

The third difficulty is that of our rapidly changing environment. We have good reason to suspect that a modern industrial society offers living conditions, such as overnutrition and physical underactivity, that are major contributors to the onset of diabetes. Yet these conditions change so rapidly that statistics based on one generation may not be applicable to the next.

It is these kinds of very practical problems that will make a full understanding of diabetic genetics extremely difficult to achieve. There is hope on the horizon, however—hope from a new discovery. Scientists have recently produced a kind of genetic "road map," which shows how all of a person's genes are put together. Thanks to this remarkable advance, there is good reason to believe that we will be able to solve the diabetic gene puzzle far sooner than previously anticipated. Meanwhile, the abnormally low incidence of the disease in the children of diabetic parents, and in the parents of diabetic children, is more than enough to suggest that we should stop torturing young diabetics with the fear of passing on the disease to their unborn children.

This returns us, finally, to the place where we began this chapter—with the story of Linda, the bright, attractive young lady who, having been coldly informed of her diabetes at age seventeen, was determined to give up all thoughts of marriage and family.

"I decided to seek psychiatric help," she told me. "After two years of therapy, I finally believed that diabetes need not be fatal. And then I met Steven. I knew after several months of dating that I cared about him very much. And he cared about me. He knew about my diabetes, but it didn't seem to matter. Soon, he proposed.

"Steven confided in me that he had doubts about having children, but after reading about diabetes, these doubts cleared up. I also spoke to my doctor about having children, and he assured me there should be no difficulty in conceiving or keeping my diabetes under control during pregnancy or delivery.

"After a year of marriage, we decided to

have a child. In my own mind, and Steven's too, I was prepared to have a healthy baby.

"Arlen Mark was four years old in April, and I still can't believe how lucky I was. Yes, it is possible for a diabetic to marry, to have children and, most of all, to lead a normal, healthy life."

6
COMPLICATIONS

NO ONE EXPECTS patients or their families to react happily to the news that they have diabetes. It is a very serious business, and must be treated accordingly. However, odd as it may sound, there *are* positive aspects to the disease, and it is important for the patient and family to know about them. It is not only unnecessary, but dangerous—physically, emotionally and psychologically—to focus constantly only on the hazards of diabetes. Nowhere is this more true than with the question of complications. We can hope that the results of the DCCT study will produce changes, but up until now the attitude of most doctors and diabetic journals toward complications has been much like the cry of "Fire!" in a crowded theater: the warning can be far more dangerous than the condition it concerns.

A positive, healthy attitude is vital to the best control of diabetes, as it is with almost any serious disease. Yet how are diabetics to attain such an outlook, when they are bombarded by frightening warnings about almost certain gangrene, amputation, blindness, heart attacks and other dreadful afflictions?

"I didn't know too much about diabetes," says Dan, an automative engineer, "but after it showed up in my medical examination, I read a couple of books about it. I wish I hadn't! Diabetes is bad enough, but all that stuff it can lead to is terrifying. The business about infection nearly wrecked me. I was afraid to leave the house because I might pick up germs or cut myself or something."

Unfortunately, such alarming books are the rule rather than the exception, even those whose titles would seem to offer help to the diabetic in adjusting to the disease. For example, when the book *Counseling and Rehabilitating the Diabetic,* by John Cull and Richard Hardy, was reviewed by the American Diabetes Association, the reviewers called the chapter on psychological adjustment to functional loss a "negative approach," which, because it equated *all* diabetes with the most crippling aspects of the disease, would "merely create or provoke anxiety."

With nothing to offset a frighteningly negative picture of the future, the diabetic and her family often react with enormous alarm to the first sign of some new "symptom"—a specific pain, for instance. When a diabetic develops neuropathy (nerve damage), it is not uncommon for the entire family, all well versed in horror stories, to accompany the patient en masse to the doctor's office to find out what dire complication this pain heralds. In actual fact, diabetic neuropathy indicates no permanent complication at all. Rather, it is connected in some still-unexplained manner with the deranged metabolism of unregulated diabetes, and heals soon after good diabetic control has been achieved and maintained. This fact notwithstanding, patients and their families are so inculcated with fear of complications that to them the pain means the certain onset of some horrible new complication—to such an extent that whenever a patient with diabetic neuropathy comes into my office, I alert my staff and household to be prepared for a slew of phone calls, local and long distance, from members of the patient's family.

Other types of pain produce similar results. I recall a very frightened twenty-six-year-old woman who consulted me in despair about her leg pains. Her mother had heard that diabetics "always lose their legs," so she was certain the pains represented the first stage of the process. In reality, they were caused by diabetic neuritis, which, although painful, disappears completely after the diabetes is brought under control. The emotional pain this young woman and her family suffered before the true situation was explained to them was totally unnecessary.

No pain was needed to frighten nineteen-year-old Ted. His fear arose from an episode of a new medical series on television. "The show was about a diabetic going blind," Ted told me, "and the doctor was using a laser to try to preserve his vision a little longer."

That program reminded Ted that he had heard a great deal about diabetics going blind. "People are always telling me about diabetic friends who've lost their eyesight. It's starting to get me up-tight. And now it's on TV. I don't think I can handle it." Typically, the television show failed to point out that the great majority of diabetics who have carefully controlled their disease suffer no visual impairment whatsoever—and that there are many medical advances available to those who do.

Television doctors, however, are not the only ones who cause unnecessary alarm. One of my patients consulted an ear, nose and throat specialist for paralysis of a vocal cord. Unable to think of any other reason for the paralysis, the doctor blamed the patient's diabetes! The real cause proved to be nothing more than overtiredness and strain. A well-regulated diabetic, such as this patient was, rarely ever develops neurologic complications . . . but the doctor found diabetes a short road to a simple answer.

Another patient of mine asked her dermatologist to inspect a lesion on her leg. The doctor asked, "Do you have diabetes?" When she acknowledged she did, he stated unequivocally, "This is a diabetic lesion." Immediately, the woman was petrified. Would she lose her leg?

The truth was that the lesion had nothing to do with the patient's diabetes; it had, in fact, been caused by varicose veins (a varicose ulcer). Even in the case of lesions that may be due in part to diabetes (ulcers of the feet, for example), there need be no serious complication if proper treatment is adhered to. But prevention is always preferable to cure, and such ulcers can be prevented through a combination of good foot care and tight control of diabetes.

Dentists, too, are often guilty of frightening patients by implying that normal dental procedures may have abnormal results in the case of the diabetic. One of my patients, for example, following extensive periodontal surgery, was told that the deterioration of his gums had been due to diabetes in the first place, and, therefore, the dentist "couldn't guarantee that the procedure would be successful.'' Neither statement was correct.

The tendency to overemphasize the importance of diabetes is commonplace among hospital personnel, a factor that adds to the distress of the diabetic patient already overwrought by whatever illness prompted his admission. A young man I know was admitted to a hospital for the diagnosis and eventual removal of a lung because of a probable lung tumor. His life was in jeopardy, but after several days of harassment by the house staff and other attendants about his diabetes control, he consulted me.

''Dr. Goodman,'' he said, ''I thought I was sent to the hospital for my lung condition. It seems like everybody here is concerned only about my diabetes, which I know is well controlled and causing me no difficulty. Why all the excitement about this? Have they forgotten why I entered the hospital?''

Why the great concern indeed? Because all of them had been taught that no medical or surgical condition will progress satisfactorily unless the diabetic patient has a normal blood sugar and negative urine tests—a goal calling for constant checks of blood and urine sugar. When, as is very often the case, this ideal state cannot be achieved, even when the diabetes is well controlled (see Chapter Three), it becomes a source of great frustration to all concerned—a frustration that cannot be hidden from an already overanxious patient.

Such fears are not limited to patients in the hospital environment. ''They say I could lose control of my diabetes even if I get just a virus of some sort,'' a young housewife told me. ''I'm not a worrywart, but that really shook me up. I know that if I lose control it could mean diabetic coma—all because I caught a virus from somebody. How do I live a normal life, with that on my mind?"

The young woman's family had been seriously affected by this concern. "Our house has become as sterile as a hospital," her husband told me. "The kids and I worry about where we go and who we see. All of us are becoming hypochondriacs. And if, God forbid, we do catch something—a sore throat, maybe—we not only worry; we feel guilty as the devil. It's hurting all of us."

Such an atmosphere can be a traumatic experience for children with a diabetic parent or sibling. They are not only deprived of a homelike environment but often are denied sympathy when they themselves become sick.

Even a constant focus on a germ-free environment is not enough to satisfy the fears of many unreasonably alarmed diabetics. "My concern is that I haven't been able to discover any concrete steps to prevent those complications I read about," one patient told me. "I've asked my doctor about this, and he says the important thing is to keep my blood sugar at the proper levels on a day-to-day basis. As long as I do this, I'm told, the complications probably won't develop. But that isn't enough. I feel I ought to be doing something specific to avoid complications. Also, I've heard that some diabetics have complications even though they do everything they're supposed to."

Such continuing frustration sometimes causes diabetics to make a complete about-face. Deciding that the onslaught of crippling complications is inevitable, they give up, throw caution to the wind and fail to heed even the most elementary rules of prevention. The result is a foregone conclusion.

The most tragic thing about all this is how utterly unnecessary such a reaction is. A physician's duty is to provide patients with enough information to cope with their future, but he or she should not be frightening them with lurid speculative descriptions. Such dire warnings serve only to make patients vulnerable to a host of imaginary ailments, while blinding them and their families to the positive aspects of their situation.

What are these aspects? In simplest terms, a diabetic may be compared to someone who has been in a serious car accident and survived. The brush with death may cause one to begin developing good safety habits involving the prevention of another accident: practicing good auto maintenance, fastening one's seat belt, staying within the speed limit, obeying other laws of the road.

In the same way, the diabetic can benefit from her disorder by developing good health habits, not only for control of her diabetes, but for her general health as well. These include sufficient rest, exercise, good foot care, a balanced diet, moderate drinking, cessation of smoking, and, perhaps most important of all, a thorough medical examination at regular intervals. Such a regimen gives the diabetic a significant health *advantage* over most other people.

Another positive aspect is that the patient and her family establish a system of contact with the doctor twenty-four hours a day, seven days a week. I instruct my patients to phone me at the first sign of any possible symptom, regardless of the hour, for I much prefer to get a telephone call at three in the morning when a problem can be treated at home or in the office than to get one at nine in the morning from the hospital emergency room. The value of such a "hot-line" system cannot be overestimated, and it gives the diabetic another significant advantage over most nondiabetics.

A final advantage is knowledge. Although all human beings ought to understand their bodies better, to know their strengths and limitations, to understand what poses a real danger and what does not, few people do. They lack the incentive to undertake such a study. The diabetic (and the diabetic's family) have that incentive.

In supplying such knowledge to my patients, I have found that it is important not only to tell them the facts about each possible area of medical complication, but also, wherever possible, to explain the background that may have led to any distorted information they received.

That is what I will do in the remainder of this chapter.

Infection

No area of possible complication is more destructive to the family life of the diabetic than fear of infection. The unnatural strain such a concern places upon the nondiabetic members of the family can result in a wide variety of psychological problems—guilt, frustration, a feeling of being unloved, anger toward the diabetic—yet no belief about possible complication is more firmly entrenched than that diabetics have a predilection to infection. The diabetic learns this early, from other patients, from books and articles, even from many doctors and nurses—yet such is *not* the case.

Authorities with the stature of Dr. M. D. Siperstein of the University of California are not only impressed with the resistance of diabetics to infection, but they state categorically that diabetics are no more susceptible to infection than other individuals. Dr. Siperstein has seen diabetics with severe ulcers of the skin come to his clinic for years without developing an infection, and he is convinced that much of the problem lies, not with any abnormal predilection to infection, but rather with something as relatively (and unfortunately) common as too-frequent catheterization of the urinary bladder.

Despite such authoritative testimony, the erroneous belief still prevails—again, the basis lies in medical history. Prior to the discovery of insulin, diabetics had good reason to fear infections: tuberculosis, for instance, was the rampant "great killer" at the turn of the century, and diabetics were particularly susceptible; carbuncles and related inflammations called furuncles (boils) were commonplace. Many other such afflictions besieged the diabetic.

Today these infections are rare, and diabetics suffer from them no more than nondiabetics. This is certainly due in part to the effective results of modern drug therapy, but there is another reason as well: the improved physical status of diabetics, as a result of insulin and other measures, has made such patients more resistant to these as well as to all other infections, with very rare exceptions.

There is a secondary basis for the diabetic's fear of infection. It is commonly thought that infection destroys the control of diabetes, thus predisposing the patient to ketoacidosis and diabetic coma and endangering his very life. He is taught that infection, trauma, stress or drugs will cause peripheral insulin resistance, which requires more insulin; that his blood sugar and insulin requirement will increase during illness; that if he doesn't meet the increased demand for insulin, he may very possibly get hyperglycemia.

To complete this terrifying picture, he is often taught that the deterioration of his diabetic control may show up initially as an elevation of the blood sugar. Thus, the moment he feels the slightest bit ill, the diabetic performs the urine or blood test and, sure enough, sees excessive glucose and acetone! He is immediately certain that he will soon wind up in the hospital.

All this is *unnecessary*. The properly informed diabetic need not be concerned about his ability to ward off loss of control and ketoacidosis in the face of illness. He need only continue taking his insulin while making certain he consumes and retains an adequate amount of carbohydrate.

If the illness produces loss of appetite or nausea, the diabetic can usually maintain his carbohydrate intake by consuming sweetened fruit juices, cold soft drinks, soup and crackers, gelatin desserts and other carbohydrates on a frequent basis. This procedure will also prevent hypoglycemic reactions.

If the patient is vomiting, the frequent consumption (every one or two hours) of high-carbohydrate drinks—orange juice, tea with sugar and so forth—will usually be sufficient, but if vomiting persists to the point where the patient is unable to retain even these liquids, then it is essential that he contact the doctor, who can see to it that glucose is administered intravenously, preferably in the hospital. This points up the importance of the hot line mentioned earlier. It is vital that the diabetic always be able to contact his physician.

My rules for diabetics who become ill can be summarized as follows:

1. Be sure to take the usual insulin injections.
2. Eat regular meals as much as possible.
3. If you are unable to eat solid food or after vomiting, take orange juice, ginger ale or other carbohydrate liquids hourly.
4. If vomiting persists, keep in constant touch with your physician.

Wound healing

Wound healing is a related problem area. Once again, many physicians are convinced that the diabetic heals poorly, and the uncontrolled diabetic even more so. Yet I have not encountered any scientific studies to substantiate this concept.

On the other hand, I *can* recall an important study by Dr. Greene of Iowa City, who compared the healing rate of surgical wounds of diabetics and nondiabetics. His study (1942) clearly showed that wounds healed as well in the diabetic as in the normal individual. Most impressive was the finding that those diabetics with the highest blood sugars healed most rapidly of all!

It is fair to state that under equivalent conditions, the diabetic can and does heal as rapidly as the normal individual.

Atherosclerosis

To the lay reader, many popularized articles appear to offer "proof" that diabetes is the cause of atherosclerosis, the underlying lesion of heart disease and stroke. The truth is, however, that atherosclerosis is the leading cause of death in the United States in *nondiabetics* as well as diabetics. Heart disease can strike anyone. To take just one example, numerous fatal heart attacks were reported from Vietnam in soldiers in their twenties, none of whom had diabetes.

The actual cause of atherosclerosis and its resultant heart disease is not yet known. Why, then, burden the diabetic and her family with the fear that diabetes will lead inevitably to a heart attack?

Without question, it is important to know that there is a statistical association between atherosclerosis and diabetes. Heart disease accounts for over half of the deaths among diabetics, and in a study of fifty thousand fatalities, coronary heart disease was reported in about twice as many diabetic as nondiabetic men and in three times as many diabetic as nondiabetic women. Thus it must be considered extremely seriously. Armed with useful information, however, the diabetic can take those measures that can help preserve her life.

First, she must maintain proper control of the diabetes. Many diabetic specialists, including myself, are firmly convinced that precise diabetic control can forestall the development of vascular lesions, and everyone agrees that *poor* control is bad. J. M. Moss found, for example, that patients in poor diabetic control showed a 10 percent decrease in longevity.

Second, the diabetic should present herself at her

doctor's office for a thorough examination at least once every year. In this way, any complication that does develop will be detected immediately and properly treated.

In sum, atherosclerosis is certainly a complication the diabetic should be careful of, but in *no* way does having diabetes mean that heart disease is inevitable; it must be remembered that atherosclerosis is the leading cause of deaths in the United States among *all* people. It picks no favorites. The diabetic who maintains excellent control of her diabetes by total adherence to her prescribed regimen of diet, exercise and "medication" and has thorough periodic examinations by the physician will help herself immeasurably. The DCCT study makes this an irrefutable conclusion.

Diabetic Neuropathy

A complication of diabetes already mentioned is nerve damage, or neuropathy. This is one of the most frequent and distressing ailments associated with diabetes, but it can be effectively treated simply by maintaining good diabetic control. Here, too, the greatest danger is from the patient's fears running rampant. Neuropathy usually strikes the lower extremities, though all the peripheral and autonomic nerves of the body are susceptible, and is characterized by destruction of the protective (myelin) sheath, which functions like the insulation of an electric light cord, leaving the nerve exposed.

The symptom that usually brings the patient to the physician is pain—pain and tingling sensations, or paresthesias, of all gradations of discomfort, from feelings of numbness, crawling on the skin and tingling, to extreme sensitivity even to the bed sheets, to steady or darting pains. All of these symptoms are worse at night, and lead the patient to envision a multitude of serious illnesses such as stroke or cancer. By the time the doctor is consulted, not only is the patient terribly agitated, but so is the entire family.

The most important thing a doctor can do at this time is to explain repeatedly to the patient and the family the nature and progress of this painful condition; to make the point that the marked discomfort is *not* caused by a fatal, serious disease but is brought on by uncontrolled diabetes; and to assure them that the nerve damage will begin to heal once good control of the diabetes has been achieved and maintained for a reasonable period.

Although the pain may last for weeks or even months, it will be handled much more easily when all concerned understand that it emanates from a benign condition—and is unlikely to bother the diabetic again so long as control is maintained.

Eyesight

Despite the clear-cut results of the DCCT study, many press releases and news articles continue to emphasize the blinding aspects of diabetes, often implying that a condition called retinopathy is inevitable if the patient has diabetes long enough. And many ophthalmologists who support the view that diabetic patients are predestined to lose their eyesight continue to maintain that good or poor control of diabetes makes no difference.

Such opinions are dangerous and based on limited or out-of-date experience. Retinopathy is by no means "predestined." The firmly held viewpoint of diabetic specialists with large clinical experience, now borne out completely by the DCCT study, is that such damage is dependent on the handling of the diabetes—the better the diabetic control, the lower the incidence and possibility of retinal lesions.

The concept that blindness was inevitable for the diabetic arose during those years before good overall control of diabetes (including diet, exercise, oral medication and insulin) was properly appreciated. During this time, it became evident to the medical profession that anatomic abnormalities were occurring in the small blood vessels of diabetics.

Put simply, diabetes is capable of damaging the capillaries in the retina, causing them to weaken and bleed. If the condition progresses, new blood vessels may form on the surface of the retina and in the vitreous humor in the center of the eye, causing further hemorrhages and blurred vision. In some cases, the blood is reabsorbed and the vision clears. In other cases, the hemorrhage causes scar tissue, which may then contract, pulling the retina, detaching or tearing it, and thereby resulting in permanent blindness.

This is a hazard that knowledgeable diabetics should very clearly understand, but they should also be aware of what the latest developments in proper diabetic care can do to prevent or delay such occurrences. Even before the DCCT, many studies strongly emphasized the importance of good diabetic control where problems involving eyesight were concerned. For instance, a twenty-five-year study reported in *The Sight-Saving Review,* involving four thousand patients and an analysis by computer of over one million pieces of information, clearly showed that retinopathy was significantly influenced by both the duration and the degree of diabetic control.

Continuous, excellent control of diabetes tends to prevent damage to capillaries. I have actually seen cases of advanced retinopathy disappear when a patient converted from poor to good diabetic control.

Even where poor control has led to retinopathy, there are many modern weapons—an amazingly wide variety of procedures—for the preservation of vision. One is the laser. An intense beam of light is directed into the retina and focused on a tiny spot, in a process that may be compared with focusing the sun's rays through a magnifying glass to burn a hole through a leaf. Heat energy generated by the light produces a small burn, which destroys the retinopathy by coagulating weakened blood vessels or destroying the proliferating vessels. If there are fragile new vessels in the treated area, they can also be destroyed, thereby preventing serious bleeding. The burn heals as a scar.

This process, called photocoagulation, was first used in 1955, so its merit has been proven over almost forty years. While vision is sometimes improved, this procedure is actually designed to prevent the more serious consequences of diabetic retinopathy and to maintain the vision at its pretreatment level. The aim is to protect the patient's most important central vision while sacrificing, if necessary, some of the less important side vision. Fortunately, the abnormal new vessels rarely grow over the essential part of the retina, called the macula, necessary for central and reading vision.

There can be no doubt that the results achieved with photocoagulation have been most rewarding, which is why the procedure is in use in clinics and hospitals and doctors' offices across the nation. In addition, the National Eye Institute is supporting a 4,000-patient, five-year clinical trial to determine new ways that photocoagulation, used alone or in combination with aspirin, can benefit people who are still in the early stages of diabetic retinopathy. This study has already proven the value of photocoagulation for macular edema and is expected to yield further valuable findings in the future.

There is also hope for those who are actually blind from massive vitreous hemorrhage or retinal detachment. Vitrectomy, a type of operation performed under the microscope, is saving the sight of some patients. As early as 1974, Dr. Guy O'Grady reported at the South Western Diabetes Symposium, sponsored by the Diabetes Association of Southern California, that he was able to produce a significant benefit in patients with a surgical device called a vitreous infusion suction cutter, developed at the Bascom Palmer Eye Institute. Resembling a large metal syringe, the extractor is powered by a small electric motor and contains three concentric tubes in its head, enabling the surgeon to incise, remove the vitreous material by suction, release bands causing retinal detachment and infuse saline solution.

Dr. O'Grady estimated that about 50 percent of the patients who were blind from diabetic retinopathy were candidates for this operation, and of the group already operated on, about half had been helped significantly.

Dr. Robert D. Reinecke, ophthalmology chairman

at Albany Medical College, said that there might be twenty-five thousand candidates for vitrectomy in the United States, including patients with end-stage diabetic retinopathy who could not be treated with laser therapy.

The results that may be achieved with this procedure were strikingly depicted in an article in the *Cleveland Plain Dealer*:

> Henry A. Gearing, 52, of Parma, is coming home tomorrow from California with newly restored vision in his left eye. Gearing has been blind for six months from blood clots in his eyes caused by diabetes. He was operated on September 30 at the Stanford University Medical Center with a new technique to remove such clots. . . . His bandages were removed 24 hours later, and it was very dramatic for him and his family. He could see. . . . He walked into the hospital with a cane and walked out last Friday with no assistance.

As dramatically impressive as these results are, I still wish to stress two points. First, diabetic patients will *not* necessarily experience any of this. Second, not even every diabetic with retinopathy need suffer visual impairment. All opthalmologists have had the happy experience of having the patient's eyesight remain good even after discovering diabetic retinopathy. Blind persons constitute a very small proportion indeed of the total diabetic population—and that is the experience of all diabetic specialists.

Like retinopathy, diabetic cataracts are written and spoken about as if they are inevitable by-products of the disease. This is not the case. They are the by-products of *uncontrolled* diabetes; they do not form without a continuing excess of blood sugar. This causes an excess of sorbitol (the alcohol of glucose) in the lens, which produces a change in the chemical balance of the lens, because the sorbitol tends to accumulate in the cells. Initially, the cataract may be detectable only through ophthalmological examination, so regular visits are a must—twice a year even if the diabetic's eyes are fine. But the point here is that these cataracts need not appear at all if the patient remembers and practices the "secrets" of continued good eyesight for the diabetic:

1. Keep control of diabetes by following the full regimen laid down by the physician.
2. Have your eyes examined twice each year, even if there are no apparent problems.
3. Keep the physician aware of any changes in the vision, no matter how small they may seem.
4. Keep a close watch on blood pressure. High blood pressure can turn minor eye problems into major ones very quickly.

Dental complications

There is a widespread belief among dentists, unfortunatetly supported by many physicians, that diabetics are taking a risk each time they visit the dentist. Even when performing essential procedures for a diabetic, procedures unhesitatingly undertaken for nondiabetics, a dentist often fears an abnormal outcome, and conveys this fear to the patient. This often causes the diabetic to postpone future visits to the dentist indefinitely and to avoid completely those very important checkups.

Yet there is no modern basis in fact for such beliefs. Some years ago, Dr. Jack Samuels and his associates undertook an impartial study in the Mount Sinai Hospital Diabetes Clinic in Cleveland, Ohio, and found that, given adequate dental attention, the diabetic was in no way more susceptible to dental ills than anyone else. The dentist—and patient—need have no fear.

Once again, control is key. Diabetics, especially Type 1 diabetics, can expect an above-average number of dental problems if they fail to exercise good control over their diabetes. Poor control may lead to gingivitis (inflamed gums) and, if this is unchecked, to periodontitis, which can destroy the bone and ligaments holding the teeth in place. When there is lack of control among juvenile diabetes, it is not uncommon to find severe periodontal disease.

None of this is necessary. The diabetic who follows a sound regimen designed to keep blood sugar close to normal, practices good dental hygiene and has regular dental checkups has no reason for concern.

Kidney damage

Kidney damage (nephropathy) is a very serious condition for diabetics and nondiabetics alike. It is found in only a small percentage of diabetics, and in a still smaller percentage of those who consistently practice good diabetic control. When the disease does occur, it presents extremely serious complications, whether the patient is diabetic or not. Its most advanced stage can result in death.

Fortunately, there are ways to guard against such dire results. Periodic testing is of great importance. Albumin in the kidney is often the first sign of kidney disease, and early testing can identify the presence of this protein. The presence of very small amounts of albumin can be detected by a simple urine test, which can be administered in the doctor's office. While this test is not foolproof evidence of kidney damage, it can be an important step in alerting you and your doctor to the need for further testing and monitoring. It can also suggest the need for changes in diet (more high protein) and stricter measures to avert or control high blood pressure.

Even if kidney disease should develop, there is still considerable room for optimism. First of all, there is the opportunity for transplant. Dr. Michall J. Kussman of the Joslin Clinic pointed out that the survival rate of diabetics with renal transplants is at least two and a half times better than that of diabetics who have suffered kidney damage but had not had transplants.

There is also dialysis, or blood filtration. At a 1974 symposium on end-stage diabetic nephropathy sponsored by the National Institute of Arthritis, Metabolism and Digestive Disease, Dr. Constantine Hampers stated that the results of dialysis on diabetic patients were immensely better than any previously reported. At the end of the first year of dialysis, over three-quarters of the juvenile-type and almost two-thirds of the adult-type diabetics had survived the procedure; compare those results with the fact that a few years earlier, diabetic kidney patients were considered too hopeless even to be put on dialysis! In addition, almost half of the patients with juvenile-type and over half of the patients with adult-onset diabetes were able to return to their jobs, a basis for rehabilitation considered very good in patients with kidney disease.

Once again, with nephropathy, as with other aspects of health, good diabetic control is a key to good health. And even for the small percentage of diabetics who do develop kidney damage, the continued advances in medical technology offer great hope.

Foot lesions

One of the pervading fears of diabetics and their families is that diabetes will lead to the loss of one or both legs. From news articles, television programs, other patients met in waiting rooms, ''helpful'' friends and relatives and even some doctors and nurses, diabetics are made to feel that the feet and legs are areas of great potential trouble. All too quickly, patients begin to envision hospitalization, loss of limb and even premature death. From this point, it is only a short step to developing a hysterical fear of venturing out of bed or a chair.

Such psychological pain is totally unnecessary, for three very good reasons. First, the loss of a limb does not occur overnight (except in the case of a sudden thrombosis, to which diabetics are no more prone than nondiabetics). It takes place in many stages, the first being the development of a diabetic foot lesion as the result of nerve damage. As we have seen, such neuropathy arises from poor diabetes control, and so the *properly* controlled diabetic should have no fear of nerve damage or foot lesions.

When nerve damage from poor control does occur, it may result in muscle imbalance that produces deformities of the toes and feet. This condition, in turn, leads to abnormal pressure on certain areas of the feet, such as the metatarsal arch, and excessive callus formation, which impinges upon the underlying skin. When these factors combine with the extreme fragility of the tissue, the groundwork is laid for skin damage and ulcer formation.

Many authorities (and much of the general public) believe that foot lesions in diabetics are the result of poor arterial circulation. This is not true. While it is a fact that many older diabetics have an inadequate blood flow in their feet as a result of atherosclerosis, this has nothing to do with lesions. In fact, there is usually quite enough flow to promote healing, provided the patient remains off his feet continuously.

The second principal reason for not worrying about foot lesions is that even for the susceptible diabetic—one who has peripheral nerve damage—such foot lesions are entirely preventable by employing proper foot hygiene (including the avoidance of too-tight shoes, going barefoot and so on) and the services of a podiatrist well versed in diabetic foot care.

The podiatrist, who can call upon training, skillful technique and experience, has the necessary expertise to prevent injury to the skin. The podiatrist who is knowledgeable about the foot problems of the diabetic trims calluses and nails—the elderly nerve-damaged diabetic should *not* trim his own toenails, corns and calluses—instructs the patient in proper foot hygiene and, when necessary, fits prostheses and special shoes to alleviate pressure in crucial areas of the feet.

Third, even if a lesion should develop on the diabetic's foot, prompt treatment brings about rapid and complete healing. In order to accomplish this, the patient must keep off his feet entirely for twenty-four hours each day, with the lesion exposed to the air. Most detrimental to the healing process in such cases is the local application of medication or ointments. Soaking the feet in hot water is absolutely forbidden.

In sum, the categorical association of diabetes and amputation is totally incorrect. The well-regulated diabetic need not sustain any nerve damage whatsoever, and so should not incur foot lesions. Where such damage has occurred, it is still possible to avoid serious foot lesions with proper foot hygiene and podiatry. And even in those cases where such lesions do exist or infection arises, complete healing can be obtained by the application of appropriate treatment.

Other medical complications

Patients who become overapprehensive about diabetes and the complications just described also tend to invent connections to all kinds of other illnesses. For instance, Bob, an otherwise well-controlled, well-adjusted diabetic, appeared at my office one morning before regular office hours. He had just been discharged from the hospital with a probable recurrence of a malignancy of the colon, which had been resected one year previously. He was receiving radiotherapy for the condition.

Two nights earlier, he had experienced a burning sensation in his tongue and found he was urinating at night every hour and a half to two hours. He interpreted these symptoms as being identical to those he

had had at the onset of his diabetes, and became
fearful that his diabetes was out of kilter. Based on
all he had heard from other diabetics, he even de-
duced that his body chemistry had been deranged by
the radiation treatments! The fact is that his symptoms were indicative of something else entirely; his
diabetes had remained perfectly controlled. In fact,
his sugar tested even better than it had six weeks
before. His concern was needless at a time when
maintaining the best possible attitude was of vital
importance.

Recently, I received a telephone call from the
daughter of a seventy-seven-year-old man who had
had to have his leg amputated, and then nearly died
from a pulmonary embolism. He had just been found
to have diabetes, but his operation was unrelated to
it. Nevertheless, when his daughter heard about the
diabetes, she became greatly alarmed, and even
though I explained that her father's diabetes was very
mild and would not harm him in the least, my words
did little to calm her fears. Because of the typical
scare stories she'd heard, she became almost as concerned about the diabetes as about her father's amputation and embolism—pointlessly, except to worry
herself.

Similarly, a patient I knew had recently returned
from the Mayo Clinic, following the removal of a
brain tumor and a subsequent prostate operation. He
had lost a lot of weight, but was getting better, and
one would have imagined that his wife, a registered
nurse, would have rejoiced at his recovery. Instead,
she became greatly perturbed by the belief that her
husband's increased food intake, necessary for post-
surgery weight gain and healing, was going to aggra-

vate his diabetes! The diabetes was actually mild and had been readily controlled without medication throughout the various hospital procedures to which he had been subjected. Still, her concern took up valuable time and energy.

At the root of this overemphasis on diabetes and other illnesses, especially in the hospital, is the opinion discussed near the opening of this chapter: that the control of diabetes is deranged by any illness. The *fact* is, the majority of diabetic patients who are admitted to the hospital with another illness have been under treatment by their physician for some time and have attained at least fairly good control. To be a well-controlled diabetic, it is not always possible, or at all necessary, to have a normal blood-sugar level and a sugar-free urine at all times. The well-controlled patient, whose blood sugar is slightly elevated and who has a modest amount of sugar in the urine, should have no difficulty whatsoever in recovering from other diseases or surgery. As a matter of fact, it is difficult for me to recall any instances of patients whose diabetes control went awry following heart attacks, infections or surgical procedures as long as there was no lapse in their regular prehospital treatment of drugs, insulin and diet. Diabetics should have no undue fear of other illness or operations.

The same is true of the other complications we have discussed in this chapter. It is important to remember that, though the diabetic can be prone to a number of complications, many of these are just as likely to happen to *nondiabetics,* and they occur only in a relatively small minority of cases. With the proper care, as recommended here and by all knowledgeable physicians and confirmed by the DCCT study, these complications, should they arise, can be kept to a minimum. In addition, given the medical technology now available, even most of those cases can be or will shortly be controlled. Don't let that cry of "Fire!" frighten you.

7

DIABETES IN CHILDREN

FORTUNATELY, DIABETES IS not a common occurrence among children (only 10 percent of recognized diabetics have Type 1, or juvenile diabetes, and only about half of these are under fifteen years of age), but when it does occur, it poses very special problems in terms of diabetic neurosis.

Obviously, any continuing illness in children carries with it great emotional stress, for both the child and the family, and this is especially true in the case of diabetes. The onset in a teenage girl or boy can be especially traumatic. Imagine the fear! And imagine how very difficult it must be for teens, who normally think of themselves as invulnerable if not immortal, to cope with the knowledge that they have a disease, that they must remain diabetics for the rest of their lives.

"Why me?" they ask, especially when informed that their whole lifestyle—what they do, what they eat, where they go—may have to change markedly. Deep feelings of guilt may get churned up, and teens may search through the past to discover what sin they have committed to merit such "punishment." In an effort to hide or overcome such guilt feelings, they may begin challenging society or blaming others, especially their parents, for their becoming diabetic. Worst of all, they may deny the presence of the disease entirely. Emotionally immature, still unsure of their identity, they may refuse to accept the reality of the medical situation and neglect their daily insulin injections or fail to follow the doctor's advice.

They may also use the disease as an excuse—a way to avoid the demands of school, social life or work—or, consciously or unconsciously, as a weapon. How many other children have such a powerful weapon to invoke against their parents, teachers or society in general? In order to get their own way or show their displeasure, they need only refuse to eat.

At a time when adolescents most wish to emulate their peers, they are constantly reminded that they are different; they must undergo daily insulin injections, blood tests and restrictions on diet; they must make special preparations for unexpected exercise; and they must guard against hypoglycemia. Even the choice of jewelry is restricted, as no ID bracelet must ever be allowed to obscure the disc that states, "I am a diabetic." For older adolescents, college and the increased independence it fosters raise additional problems. Decisions concerning such common occurrences as drinking, for instance, can be especially difficult.

Parental concern, although of quite a different nature, is just as strong. The following, from a father who discovered that his child had diabetes, is a typical sentiment:

The doctor must have been looking at us rather closely as my wife and I sat in his office expecting the worst and then hearing our suspicions clearly confirmed. I'm sure that neither of us knew exactly what we were thinking at that moment, for it was a jolt. . . . We had thought this might be the case but had desperately hoped it would not be. Now, suddenly, we had this totally new situation on our hands, which neither of us was ready, willing or able to cope with.

Of course, the doctor (who had delivered all four of our sons) was trying to assure us that the end of the world had not yet arrived and Larry could live a normal life. He had never deceived us, and I suppose this should have been enough to allay our fears, but it wasn't. It didn't even begin to untie the anxious knot in the pit of my stomach.

After the initial shock wore off and I began to use more reason and less emotion, I learned that the local hospital was giving a course in the basics of diabetes for the benefit of juvenile diabetics and, more important, for their parents.

At the first meeting, I thought I'd confused the room numbers and was at a session of Alcoholics Anonymous. It was awful. One of the first things the doctor asked of that rather shy group in attendance was, "How many of you are diabetics?" Just as straight out as that! I watched my twelve-year-old son rather timidly raise his hand to about half-mast and mentally countered: "What a way to start a class on diabetes."

Then it really hit me—not only because my son had diabetes and I was scared silly as to how he would make out in school all by himself, but also because I had been teaching for almost thirty years, and I didn't have the foggiest idea what I would, could or even should do if one of my students had an insulin reaction. If I didn't know, how many other teachers would?

Fearful parents augment the emotional problems of their diabetic child in ways both subtle and overt. The cycle often begins when someone attempts to establish whether heredity can explain the reason for the child's disease. Though the only familial connection may be old Uncle John, who had diabetes when he died at age eighty-two, this remote connection is sufficient to supply a source for guilt.

Another and more potent source of guilt comes when the mother is questioned about her pregnancy. She often becomes convinced that she must have made errors, especially in her diet, while carrying the child, and now tries to redeem herself by constant and excessively careful surveillance of the child's meals. As her diabetic offspring becomes the focus of attention, desserts for all family members begin to disappear, life becomes more regimented and family closeness often disintegrates. Hostilities that had been dormant suddenly emerge like ants swarming around sugar.

Nor is the family's peace of mind improved by information gleaned from other diabetics or even from "expert" commentary printed in various publications. The following statement from a Cleveland newspaper was made by the president of a local chapter of the National Juvenile Diabetic Foundation, an organization charged with the responsibility of *improving* the lot of diabetic children and their parents:

They get their children up in the morning, give them insulin shots, see them off to school with their tags in place, their special candy in their pockets.

The candy is not a treat. It is meant to save the child's life if the body chemistry goes awry.

The tags are not jewelry. They are worn to alert a stranger who could find the child in insulin shock.

For the mother of the diabetic child, life is a constant worry, a constant watching for telltale signs of trouble.

She knows it is important for him to lead as normal a life as possible, but she knows also that there is a tragic difference between her child and the child next door.

Yet, when diabetes is found in a child, the reaction on the part of friends and relatives is usually, "Just be thankful that it is not a serious disease."

"What could be more serious?" asked Mrs. George Hawk, president of the local chapter of the National Juvenile Diabetes Foundation and the mother of a four-year-old diabetic. "Our children usually live only a short life after the disease is discovered in them. They face blindness, severe kidney damage, the loss of their legs."

Diabetes is the fifth leading cause of death in the country.

Imagine the parents of a diabetic child reading such a news item without any other information about diabetes to offset it! The damage to family morale caused by such totally unwarranted, unbalanced articles is all too obvious.

PREMATURE AGING LINKED TO DIABETES

This alarming headline, printed in a Cleveland daily newspaper, is another example of the type of writing that can be so injurious to the diabetic child and his family. The news item was based on an article by Dr. Robert H. Kohn, professor of pathology at Case Western Reserve University Medical School. Dr. Kohn stated that severe diabetes starting in childhood may cause an accelerated aging of important connective tissue in the body, making the young old before their time; and he described connective tissue resembling that of people aged eighty-four and one hundred and six appearing in patients whose actual ages were thirty-three and forty-four.

Such an article never should have been printed, for Dr. Kohn himself acknowledged that the three diabetic cases were only a small part of a long-term study of aging, and that the data were inconclusive and did *not* prove that the described changes were the result of diabetes. The fact of the matter is, nondiabetics *also* experience the greatest increase in stiffness of the connective tissue between the ages of thirty and fifty.

The list of such misleading published statements goes on and on. Consider this one in the *American Medical News* by Dr. Arthur Rubinstein:

> Diabetes, though ''manageable'' in most adult victims, takes on a grimmer aspect when it strikes children. Though the one-million-plus juvenile diabetics can buy time with insulin and regular care, there is no tangible hope of a cure or a way to head off the more serious complications in later life.
>
> Young diabetics should be told the truth. It's self-defeating not to in the long run, since for the time being there isn't a thing we can do about it.

Very well. Let us tell young diabetics the facts. But is this bleak, depressing picture really the truth? I have never believed it. And, finally, the recent DCCT study has provided conclusive proof that such pessimistic prose is entirely unwarranted. With optimal treatment, diabetes need not disable children or hinder their activity. Diabetic children grow normally, attend school, get married and raise families like anyone else. They are able to attend college and participate in athletics and leisure activities. Upon completion of schooling, they hold positions in keeping with their abilities, and they live to ages comparable to those attained by other healthy children.

These are the facts. But the key to all of this is proper treatment. Let's look now at the diabetic child and see how diabetes for her or him differs from that of most adults—and how this diabetes can best be treated.

Insulin

Insulin is almost always essential to the control of diabetes in children. Even if, as sometimes happens, there is a brief period of remission when insulin *could* be discontinued, the physician is wise to continue at least "token" injections during this period. Dr. Stuart Carne explains why:

> In a very few children, there may be a period, usually shortly after initial diagnosis has been made, when control of the diabetes appears to be satisfactory without insulin, but almost always this "honeymoon" period is brief and the need for insulin soon reappears. It is, therefore, unfair in such cases to discontinue the insulin, however little the quantity needed, because the psychological trauma of having to resume injections may be worse than the advantage of temporarily stopping them.
>
> There are extremely few children (perhaps only a handful recorded in the world medical literature) with proven diabetes in whom there is any lengthy period of freedom from the need for insulin.

In other words, once the child has adjusted to the idea of daily injections, halting them—something that would almost certainly be a temporary measure— would give the child unwarranted reason to believe the diabetes was improving, that injections might never be needed again. Subsequent return to the injections could be traumatic.

Diabetes in children is characterized by marked rises and sudden precipitous drops in blood sugar, changes that range from perhaps 70 mg percent to 500 mg percent. Because of such fluctuations, the diabetic child is more prone than most adult diabetics to hypoglycemia (insulin reaction), and should be taught to recognize the symptoms—declining academic performance, unusual fatigue, inability to concentrate, inattention, behavioral problems—and to overcome them quickly by eating something. The child's teachers should also be alert to the symptoms and bring them promptly to the attention of the school nurse and the parents.

Hypoglycemia can be treated by administering sugar in one of many forms. If the child is awake and cooperative, he or she can be given several sugar cubes, fruit juice with added sugar (a glass of orange juice with one or two tablespoons of sugar) or regular carbonated beverages or candy (not diet or ''dietetic''). The symptoms should clear in ten or fifteen minutes.

If the child is irrational, combative, semiconscious or unconscious, food or fluids should not be forced. Instead the child should be taken to the nearest hospital emergency room, where intravenous glucose or glucagon can be administered. Drugs such as glucagon (for injection) are also available for administration by parents, but only by prescription. These drugs have some built-in dangers and are generally prescribed only for children who have a history of sudden hypoglycemia leading to unconsciousness. Even in these cases, prevention—extremely careful control of blood sugar—is a far better approach. In other words, care should be taken to stop hypoglycemia *before* it starts.

Dr. G. D. Molnar in an *International Medical News* article stressed that insulin overdosage is the most significant cause of hypoglycemia in the young diabetic, and, as we have seen, this overdosage is very often the result of mistaken attempts to achieve and maintain sugar-free blood tests. Such attempts are not only unrealistic but dangerous. For the best diabetic control, it is frequently necessary to compromise the strict blood-sugar standards many doctors have promulgated. "With some patients," Dr. H. C. Knowles pointed out in that same article, "you have to tolerate higher sugar levels." And still another diabetes expert, Dr. R. F. Bradley, concurred in that same article, readily admitting that some sugar is often an acceptable and realistic result of treatment.

Multiple doses (rather than a single daily injection) are essential in developing and maintaining control. Long before the DCCT study, many diabetic authorities agreed that this is the most successful treatment for a juvenile diabetic. Such a regimen may be difficult for some schedules, but it has the extra advantage of stimulating the action of the normal pancreatic cells and permitting the lowest possible total dose of insulin. In the beginning, I start patients on regular insulin because its effect is most predictable, but I usually find it necessary later to add an intermediate-acting insulin (Lente or NPH) to one or more doses.

Whatever the method used by the physician, one fact stands out: every diabetic has an individual dosage that is best for him or her. It is the doctor's responsibility to find this dosage and carefully tailor the prescription to the patient's special requirements.

Before we leave the subject of insulin, one last word about the child's responsibility. Since insulin is a major factor in the treatment of diabetes, it is very important that the child be instructed by his physician in the use of insulin soon after the disease is diagnosed, even if he is too young yet to give himself injections. Diabetic children should learn about the insulin's importance to the body, the proper method of administration, the amount and type to give and where to inject it. By the time they are ten years of age, many children are able to administer insulin properly to themselves.

Diet and exercise

Young people with diabetes face many challenges but also have the same basic requirements, both physical and emotional, that other children share. Their diet, for example, must be designed to meet all their needs for growth, maturation and the varying energy requirements of childhood. In most cases, the school lunch program is acceptable for the noon meal.

The most important thing to remember is that the energy value of the overall diet must be designed so that children attain and then maintain an ideal body weight. In fact, the optimum diet for the young diabetic is so well balanced that the entire family could take note of it. A family with a diabetic child often finds that overall nutrition is *improved* after it adopts the basic pattern recommended for the patient!

As for sports, there is no reason why diabetic chil-

their own needs and those of any other children in the family. The key to good health for the diabetic child is good health for the entire family. With this in mind, many parents join support groups. The physician or the nearest office of the American Diabetes Association can provide families with the address and phone number of the nearest support group.

A frank, objective talk with a doctor who is not emotionally involved with the family can eliminate many of the fantasies children may have, fantasies promoted by the parents' guilt and their need to conceal their feelings. The physician should explain to both the children and their families the history of the disease and its misapprehensions: that its cause is unknown; that the symptoms result from an insulin deficiency; and that with insulin available, the disorder can be overcome so that the body functions normally. Adolescent patients typically welcome honesty and nonjudgmental discussions with the physician. Given the right kind of guidance, their diabetes can even be a *positive impetus* toward growth and maturity.

Today's diabetic child is permitted all the food other children eat, and he or she grows like anyone else. The fear of severe dietary restrictions can be forgotten (see Chapter Four). In order for things to go smoothly, however, there are a few inconveniences: careful monitoring and regimen-following at home, and regular visits to the doctor's office, so that the diabetes can be observed closely and adjustments made when necessary.

Dr. E. Podell has summarized very well the proper

approach to diabetes in children and adolescents in *Medical Insight:*

1. Establish goals based on reality, not fantasy.
2. Provide total education about diabetes. The young diabetic must be familiar with every aspect of diabetes, and the educational process should include results of the latest research.
3. Establish self-responsibility as soon as possible. This should go beyond simply the self-administration of insulin and should also include the responsibility for purchasing and caring for insulin and syringes.
4. Provide an adult figure, who is not involved with the child's everyday life, to whom he or she can relate. The physician can certainly be this person, and his support and counseling can greatly enhance the adolescent's emotional stability. The physician needs to establish confidentiality and still be able to involve the total family when conflicts are related to parent-child relationships.
5. Recognize the importance of the child's peer relationships. Healthy friendships (and antagonisms) allow diabetic adolescents to work out mood swings and identify their causes.
6. Consider the realities of the frequent change in life-style. *Change* is one word that can be used universally to describe the world of the adolescent.

A great deal of credit is due the mothers and fathers who are forthright with their children and assist in their learning to accept diabetes. Diabetic children who make a good adjustment reflect the healthy attitudes of their parents, and children are fortunate if their parents, having learned to handle their own concerns in this matter, support their children well. The discipline learned at home will help them develop into mature, responsible people who will be able to take pride in their ability to manage their own health problems successfully.

Overprotection

Even the most well-intentioned parents find it difficult to avoid displaying at least some measure of overprotectiveness toward the diabetic child. In addition, the very idea of being "sick" can make some children feel less capable than their friends, so special efforts should be made to develop their sense of independence.

I particularly recommend the use of camps for diabetic children, whenever they are available (see the Appendix). As R. K. McGray and L. B. Travis found when they evaluated a group of children with diabetes before and after attending a special camp, those who attended one showed a marked increase in their self-esteem and a heartening decrease in anxiety.

In some camps, the youngsters are encouraged to maintain their own tents and cook their own meals. They take canoe trips on rivers, an undertaking that might have posed a threat for diabetics some years ago but is now made practical by the availability of a wide variety of light, easily transportable foods, which provide the essential nutrients needed to meet even the strictest diet requirements.

Other camps take their charges to the top of high mountains, proving to the climbers that, within reason, they can do anything others can do. "The words 'I can't' are never permitted in our camp," says one director. "All too often in real life, teenagers defeat themselves before tackling something."

The values delivered by special diabetes camps are well summarized by the father of a child who attended one: "I believe that my wife and I had a feeling somewhat akin to Hannibal at the crest of the Alps when we sent Larry to camp for a week last summer. He sailed through one week of activities without a problem, all on his own, without help from anyone! This was a direct result of the training he received, and it taught him more about the fact that a diabetic can and should follow a normal life than anything he could read or hear."

8

RESEARCH ON DIABETES

RESEARCH PROGRAMS CURRENTLY underway and
likely to bear fruit within the next few years offer
more reasons for a positive attitude on the part of
diabetics and their families. Progress can be seen in
a multitude of areas, such as more effective delivery
of insulin, predicting the likelihood of diabetes, prevention of the disease and its cure. Let us look briefly
at some of this research.

Cause, Cure and Concern

Considerable work is being done with antibodies in
an effort to predict diabetes. This will not only help
those most susceptible do what they can to slow or
prevent the onset of the disease; it will also help
researchers gather data that should eventually lead to
uncovering the cause and cure of diabetes.

Already this research has produced the islet-cell
antibody test. When the immune system begins destroying the beta cells of the pancreas, the islet-cell
antibody shows up in the bloodstream. This antibody

appears well ahead of the time when the blood-sugar level shoots up, so it is a very early indication that diabetes (Type 1) has begun to develop.

Using this test, siblings, parents or children of diabetics can determine whether the disease is developing in their bodies. This is particularly helpful to those who experience diabetic neurosis out of intense concern that "heredity" may cause them or their children to develop the disease.

"Even five years ago, no one thought it would ever be possible to prevent diabetes," says Dr. Richard A. Jackson, head of the Hood Center for Prevention of Childhood Diabetes at the Joslin Diabetes Center in Boston, "but today we can already prevent Type 1 diabetes in animals prone to developing the illness. And my pilot study with humans has made me optimistic."

What was Dr. Jackson's recent pilot study? He examined twelve close relatives of patients with Type 1 diabetes; blood tests of all twelve revealed islet-cell antibodies. He treated five of these with small doses of insulin "to give the remaining beta cells a rest and prevent their collapse." Only one of those five developed diabetes. The other seven relatives turned down the therapy. *All seven eventually developed diabetes!*

As of June 1994, eighty thousand people are in the process of being screened in order to find four hundred with higher-than-average risk for Type 1 diabetes. They will then be recruited for a research project designed to provide statistical proof that the conclusions drawn from Dr. Jackson's pilot study are (or are not) accurate.

Transplant

The first success with the transplant of a pancreas dates back more than thirty years, yet there has been far less progress in this area than might be expected. Why? The initial enthusiasm for the transplant work pioneered by Drs. DeJode and Howard in 1963 was relatively short-lived. Although some twenty-three transplants had been performed in the next seven years, patients died of various causes soon after the operation. The longest anyone survived was only a little over a year.

The basic problem with transplanting the pancreas was summarized very succinctly by Dr. H. T. Ricketts in an article published in 1974: "The success of immunology has not advanced far enough to guarantee against rejection." Twenty years later, that statement remains true. In some organs—the heart, for example—problems can be matters of life and death, justifying the risk of transplant rejection; in the pancreas, however, problems can generally be handled quite well by means other than transplanting. Thus, progress in this field has not occurred at the rate one might otherwise anticipate.

Nevertheless, some advances have been made. Length of survival for patients after transplant has improved, and the "new" pancreas often produces insulin for a longer period of time. And there is promise in the work with islet cells. The transplanting of these cells has suffered the same rate of rejection as that for the total pancreas, but various materials that would apply a "coating" to the cells, giving them "armor" to protect against rejection by the body, are now being tested.

Insulin Pumps

With the DCCT study finally providing conclusive proof of the value of tight control, there is increased demand for simplification of the means of maintaining that control—in particular, for a method of delivering insulin as needed without multiple injections each day. This increase in demand will very likely lead to a speedup of research in an area that has, until now, moved with disappointing languor.

Currently, the apparatus used most widely is the "open-loop" insulin pump, one that delivers a constant low-level supply but cannot measure the body's increased need for insulin (after meals, for example), so it must be adjusted by the wearer. Aside from not being automatic, these open-loop pumps have the added negatives of high cost ($2,000–$3,000) and the fact that wearing a device plugged into one's stomach is a constant reminder of the presence of diabetes—a reminder that can also become painful if infection develops at the hookup site, something that is not unusual. This is a machine, of course, and mechanical failings have caused severe insulin reaction and other problems. My recommendation, except in very special circumstances, is that patients should avoid the pump for the time being. Researchers are working on improvements, however, and the hope is that these machines will be much better in the near future.

"Closed-loop" pumps—those that can detect changes in blood glucose and adjust the insulin delivery *automatically*—are thus far limited primarily to hospitals because of their size (they are consoles) and complexity. But various miniaturized, implantable versions are already being tested, and the growing

DCCT-fostered desire for easier, more efficient delivery systems should accelerate the research and produce meaningful results very soon.

The Eyes

As mentioned in Chapter Six, the National Eye Institute is supporting a nationwide study to determine to what degree photocoagulation, used alone or in combination with aspirin, can benefit people who are still in the early stages of diabetes retinopathy. Almost four thousand patients are enrolled in this five-year clinical trial, which has already proven the value of photocoagulation for macular edema and is expected to deliver further valuable findings in the near future.

In addition to these trials, the Institute is supporting an extensive program of research on the causes, detection and treatment of retinopathy.

Other Research

Research advances important for diabetics are also being made in less directly related fields. Genetic researchers, for example, are working on producing a sort of "map" that shows how all of a person's genes fit together—which should lead to the discovery of the gene related to diabetes. The potential value of this discovery cannot be overestimated.

Advances in food research are also significant. The discovery that carbohydrates with similar numbers of calories and nutrients are absorbed into the blood at different rates of speed (and therefore have different effects on blood sugar) is already leading to increased glucose control via diet.

In the years since the first edition of this book was printed, two totally different areas of research have been brought to fulfillment: the development of a small, portable device for testing blood-glucose levels at home, and the DCCT study that has proved the tremendous value of proper diabetes control.

Consider first what these advances mean *today* in terms of improvement for the diabetic's life. And then consider how such advances will accelerate research in other areas! Clearly, the future—both immediate and long-range—looks bright for the diabetic.

9

THE POSITIVE APPROACH

PROPER DIABETIC EDUCATION is essential if diabetics and their families are to be able to understand and then to ignore the scare stories on the subject in articles, books, TV shows and Hollywood movies. Only through such education can diabetics and their loved ones avoid or overcome diabetic neurosis, and only in this way can they develop the affirmative approach so vital to proper care and treatment of the disease.

As we have seen, diabetes is best controlled not by fear and dread, but by knowledge and self-assurance—by a positive attitude.

The advantages of such an attitude may become clear through the following example. In the course of my medical practice, I have encountered many patients with insomnia. Most tend to complain about their sleeplessness, about the fact that they are unable to enjoy the same amount of rest as other members of their household, but others—I recall one in particular—have turned the disability to their advantage instead. Recognizing that for some unexplained reason they simply cannot sleep as long as most people, they take those hours of solitude and use them to gain extra knowledge. One automobile executive told me quite frankly that he considered his insomnia to be "the secret of my success."

In much the same way, diabetes can be one's "secret of success" in terms of a healthy, happy life. If diabetic patients accept the reality of the disease rather than fight it, if they use it as a barometric enforcer of good health, they will find themselves turning a negative into a positive.

Dr. L. Matthews, professor of pediatrics at Case Western Reserve University, whom we first met in Chapter One, expressed this very well:

> So you have diabetes? Is that so bad? I don't think so, and I feel I should know, since I've had diabetes since 1957. If one had a choice, I'm certain we would all choose perfect health. But if one has to have a chronic disease, and we really have no choice, then I feel we are fortunate to have diabetes.
>
> I found it possible to achieve every goal I set for myself in academic pediatrics, to raise a family of five energetic children, to paint my own home, to wallpaper every room of it, to be a family traveler and camper, and even extend the lives of my cystic fibrosis patients, some of whom have diabetes in addition to cystic fibrosis.
>
> I write this only to attempt to convince you that having diabetes can even be an advantage. It's a disease you don't have to be ashamed of, one you can even be proud to have conquered.

Don't hide it or use it as an excuse. Use it as an increased incentive.

E. Hill, a diabetic of many years, presented much the same viewpoint in his 1974 article for the *Diabetes Newsletter,* published by the Diabetes Association of Greater Cleveland:

> When someone asks what kind of problem I have with diabetes, I usually reply that the only problem I have is in thinking of a problem when asked. Having reached the age of twenty-three after twenty-one years of diabetes, my life is as active and full as that of any of my fraternity chums who have a reputation of being the most active students at the dental school.
>
> My diabetes has not prevented me from achieving everything I have wanted to accomplish, and I see no reason for that condition to change.

More recently, actor Wilford Brimley said, "If I keep control and do what I've been told to do, then I expect that I will live a long and healthy life—maybe longer than it would have been if diabetes hadn't caused me to start taking better care of myself."

Such positive attitudes can be instilled in children at a very early age. Danny had been under my care for two years at the time of this story. From the beginning, his parents had accepted the disease fully, and Danny had no trepidation whatsoever about his diabetes. During the summer of his ninth year, he spent two full weeks at a summer camp. This was not a camp for diabetics; accordingly, Danny had to administer his own insulin and eat the regular camp food. The result: a wonderful time. As one might expect, Danny returned home in the best of health and spirits and with a renewed sense of self-assurance.

Some time ago, the father of two teenage diabetic daughters, who had received their diagnoses within two weeks of each other, phoned to inquire about a minor ailment one of them had. During the conversation, he expressed his appreciation for the care given his daughters. He pointed out that following their diagnoses, they had walked around completely bewildered, their heads bowed, but after receiving a clearer, more comprehensive picture of their disease and their future lives, they had perked up rapidly and become once again two normal, happy girls.

This kind of positive acceptance can be used as an example for adults as well. A thirty-year-old woman who was unable to accept the fact of her diabetes was counseled on the subject by a young nurse who had lived with diabetes since the age of nine. The nurse pointed out that if a nine-year-old child and her family could adjust to and accept diabetes well enough to raise that child and send her happily into a nursing career, then why couldn't a mature, thirty-year-old woman make the same sort of adjustment? The woman made a complete about-face in her attitude.

The positive attitudes of well-adjusted diabetics are best expressed in the words of the patients themselves. Here, for example, is a bit of tennis great Bill Talbert's story of his youth:

I was ten years old when my illness began. I would come home from school and plop into bed, almost too tired to raise my head. I gulped down water as if I were marooned on a desert island. I ate as if food was going to be outlawed. I went to the bathroom too often.

My mother and father took me to the doctor. I had diabetes. Not too many years before, there'd been nothing for a diabetic to do but waste away and ultimately die. The discovery of insulin had brightened the overall picture, but the diabetic's fate was inactivity. Baseball was out. No more sports of any kind for me—until that day Dad came home with a package under his arm.

"What's that?" my mother asked.

"A tennis racket for Billy," said my father.

My mother was visibly upset. "You're not going to let that boy play tennis, are you?" she inquired, incredulous.

I was fourteen then. My dreams of baseball dashed, I was happy to play any sport—even a sissy game like tennis.

Bill Talbert did play that "sissy" game. He went on to become one of the world's best-known tennis champions, winning the National Men's Doubles Championship (four times), the National Men's Indoor Doubles (four times), the National Men's Indoor Singles (twice) and the Clay Court Singles. Later, Bill Talbert became a highly successful executive for the Security–Columbian Banknote Company of New York.

Ron Santo, a remarkably gifted baseball player

who played for both the Chicago White Sox and the Cubs, discovered he was a diabetic when he was just nineteen. Quoted in *Sports-Medicine,* he said:

When you consider all the diseases that can't be controlled, it's almost a relief to have diabetes. I eat just about anything I want. I haven't had any complications. I've had operations and injuries—my jaw busted, a broken wrist, cuts— and they all healed well because I have taken very good care of myself. I've never been in a coma.

For the first five years I had diabetes, I pretty much kept it to myself. But after I made a couple of All-Star teams and felt I was becoming established, I told the club's physician, Dr. Jacob Suker, and the organization. Even then I kept it quiet for a while, but eventually I made a point of talking to groups of kids who had diabetes, and to their parents. I tried to give them my side of the story, which is, "Sure, diabetes is a disease, but it's a disease you can handle if you just make an effort."

My life's been no different from anybody else's. The shots to me are nothing. They're my normal routine—like waking up and putting on my pants. It's not a disease you can take lightly, and if you don't accept it, you are going to have problems. But if you know what it's all about, you can live a full, healthy life.

Bruce Taylor is not a celebrity, but the words of this young man seem very appropriate here:

One day I learned that a friend of my father's had cancer of the stomach. Knowing that I was a diabetic, he said that he would give anything if he could have injections every day to control his disease. What he said punctured my balloon of self-pity. I realized that if it were not for insulin, I would be dead.

Before insulin was first discovered by Drs. Banting and Best, I would have been put on a starvation diet and had a life expectancy of a few months to—at most—a few years. I began to see how lucky I was after all those days when I had simply accepted life, never giving a thought as to how beautifully such a complex machine as the human body works.

Insulin. That one word is now synonymous with life. Now every day that I am able to live is indeed a special day. I keep thinking whenever I hear of someone with cancer, "What would he give if he could have injections every day that would alleviate his disease so that he could lead a normal life?"

What would you give if you were blind and found that by taking injections each day you could see? What would you give? Or ask yourself what can one give for all the courage, time, energy, experiments, failures, successes which some people face so that someone else may live—someone like me, whom Dr. Banting and Dr. Best never met or ever will meet?

Thanks. I worship life. Every minute. When I became a diabetic and then realized how lucky I was to still be alive, I began to see how incredibly beautiful the world is. From then on, whenever I saw a wave kiss the shore or watched a sunset, my reaction was no longer, "Gee, isn't that nice." Instead, it was, "My God! I'm alive to see all this!"

And when I saw a person suffering, I no longer said, "Gee, that's too bad," but rather, "What can I do to help?" That's why I worked for my degree in sociology from the University of Washington. And that's why I have begun to write. Perhaps there is something I can do or say that will help others. Perhaps these words have given someone, somewhere, something that he or she did not have before. It may be hope, for that is what I feel—hope and faith in the future. Hope and faith in humanity. The nobility of mankind seeking answers, never satisfied—striving, conquering, healing.

No, no. I will not be resentful of diabetes again. I have learned too much. I have learned not only how beautiful life is but what it means to live. I have learned how to make every minute count, how to regard every flower as a universe within itself, how to regard life as a universe.

That is what diabetes taught me. It has caused a new awareness in my life. Although being a diabetic has its complications, the fact that I live—that I have life—far outweighs any detrimental factor.

Now I know how valuable life is.

As I reach the end of this book, it seems fitting to return to the beginning—to the words of Mary Tyler

Moore, one of television's most talented and successful actresses.

"The most amazing thing about diabetes," said Ms. Moore, "is the complete lack of knowledge that exists about it. When I first learned I had it, I was very frightened. I wondered, 'Am I going to be an invalid? Will I be bedridden?' I just didn't know."

But Mary Tyler Moore went on to find out. She learned about diabetes—learned how to care for it and how to make it work for her.

"I check in with my doctor much more than the average person does," the actress explains. "He can spot trouble in other areas long before the average person is going to spot it, because the average person might go to his doctor only once or twice a year. I go at least four or five times a year."

Finally, Ms. Moore offers some words of inspiration for all diabetics and their families: "Maybe it isn't a blessing to be a diabetic, but people who find out they have diabetes can easily turn what might appear to be a negative into a very important positive. I know that I did."

And you can, too.

APPENDIX:

Summer Camps for Diabetic Children

THE FOLLOWING IS a list of fifty-one summer camps for children with diabetes that are sponsored by the American Diabetes Association.

ARIZONA

Camp Azda

Arthur Talbot
ADA Arizona Affiliate
2328 W. Royal Palm Road,
Suite D
Phoenix, AZ 85021
602-995-1515

CALIFORNIA

Bearskin Meadow Camp

Ronald Brown
Diabetic Youth
Foundation

1954 Mt. Diablo
Boulevard, Suite A
Walnut Creek, CA 94596
510-937-3393

Camp Chinnock

Joanie Johnston
ADA California Affiliate
10445 Old Placerville
Road
Sacramento, CA 95827
916-369-0999

Camp De Los Ninos

Madelyn Zelman
Santa Clara Valley
Diabetes Society

1261 Lincoln Avenue,
#208
San Jose, CA 95125
408-287-3785

COLORADO

Children's Diabetes Camp

Browning Lummus
ADA Colorado Affiliate
2450 S. Downing
Denver, CO 80210
303-778-7556

CONNECTICUT

Youth Summer Camp Program

Liana Desroches
ADA Connecticut
Affiliate
300 Research Parkway
Meriden, CT 06450
203-639-0385

FLORIDA

Florida Camp For Children and Youth

Rosalee Bandyopadhyay
PO Box 14135,
University Station
Gainesville, FL 32604
904-392-4123

GEORGIA

Camp Liwidia

Todd Garrett
ADA Georgia Affiliate
3782 Presidential Park-
way, Suite 102
Atlanta, GA 30340
404-454-8401

ILLINOIS

Camp Granada

Donna Scott
ADA Downstate Illinois
Affiliate
2580 Federal Drive
Decatur, IL 62526
217-875-9011

Teen Adventure Camp

Mary Delacey
ADA Northern Illinois
Affiliate
6 N. Michigan Avenue,
Suite 1202
Chicago, IL 60602
312-346-1805

YMCA Camp Duncan

Suzanne Apsey
ADA Northern Illinois
Affiliate
6 N. Michigan Avenue,
Suite 1202
Chicago, IL 60602
312-346-1805

INDIANA

Camp John Warvel

Elaine McClane
ADA Indiana Affiliate
222 S. Downey Avenue
Indianapolis, IN 46219
317-352-9226

IOWA

Camp Hertko Hollow

Beth Volz
ADA Iowa Affiliate
6656 Douglas Avenue
Des Moines, IA 50322
515-276-2237

KANSAS

Camp Discovery

Bonnie Simon
ADA Kansas Affiliate
3210 E. Douglas
Wichita, KS 67208
316-684-6091

LOUISIANA

La Lions Camp For Youth with Diabetes

Becky Day
ADA Louisiana Affiliate
9420 Lindale Avenue,
Suite B
Baton Rouge, LA 70815
504-927-7732

MAINE

Camp Kee-to-Kin

Joan MacCraken, MD
Eastern Maine Medical
Center
489 State Street
Bangor, ME 04401-6674

MARYLAND

Camp Glyndon

ADA Maryland Affiliate
2 Reservoir Circle,
Suite 203
Baltimore, MD 21208
410-486-5515

MASSACHUSETTS

Clara Barton Camp For Girls with Diabetes

Kassie Gregorio
68 Clara Barton Road,
Box 356
North Oxford, MA 01537
508-987-2056

Elliott J. Joslin Camp For Boys with Diabetes

Paul Madden
Joslin Diabetes Center
One Joslin Place
Boston, MA 02215

MICHIGAN

Camp Midicha

Ann Patronik
ADA Michigan Affiliate
23100 Providence Drive,
Suite 400
Southfield, MI 48075
313-552-0480

Camp Midicha-UP

Ann Patronik
ADA Michigan Affiliate
23100 Providence Drive,
Suite 400
Southfield, MI 48075
313-552-0480

MISSISSIPPI

Twin Lakes Camp '93

Mary Forturne
ADA Mississippi Affiliate
16 Northtown Drive,
S-100
Jackson, MS 39211
601-957-7878

MISSOURI

Camp Edi

ADA Missouri Affiliate
1316 Parkade Boulevard
PO Box 1013
Columbia, MO 65205
314-443-8611

Camp Shawnee

ADA Missouri Affiliate
1316 Parkade Boulevard
PO Box 1013
Columbia, MO 65205
314-443-8611

Camp Red-Bird

Stephanie Tranen, MPH,
RD
American Diabetes
Association
9440 Manchester Road,
Suite 104
St. Louis, MO 63119
314-968-3196

MONTANA

Camp Diamont

Stanlee Dull
ADA Montana Affiliate
Box 241I
Great Falls, MT 59403
406-761-0908

NEW HAMPSHIRE

Camp Carefree

Robbi Conley
ADA New Hampshire
Affiliate
104 Middle Street
Manchester, NH 03101
603-627-9579

NEW JERSEY

Camp Nejeda

Janice Burd
Saddleback Road
PO Box 156
Stillwater, NJ 07875-0156
201-383-2611

NEW YORK

Camp Sunshine

Beverly Gaines
American Diabetes
Association
1650 Elmwood Avenue
Rochester, NY 14620
716-271-1260

NORTH CAROLINA

Camp Carolina Trails

Jennifer Lamm
2315-A Sunset Avenue
Rocky Mount, NC 27804
919-937-4121

NORTH DAKOTA

Camp Sioux

Susan Weaver
ADA North Dakota
Affiliate
101 N. 3rd Street,
Suite 400
Grand Forks, ND 58203
701-746-4427

OHIO

Camp Korelitz

Kevin Vance
3605 Pape Avenue
Cincinnati, OH 45208
513-281-0002

OKLAHOMA

Camp Ne Oca Da

Phyllis Raines
American Diabetes
Association
7230 E. 64th Place
Tulsa, OK 74133
918-492-5828

Camp O'Leary/ Kno-Keto

Darrell Smith
ADA Oklahoma Affiliate
3909 Classen Boulevard, #101
Oklahoma City, OK 73118
405-525-0222

Camp Red-Bud

Denny Krick, ED.D.
Garfield County Health Department
2501 Mercer Drive
Enid, OK 73701
405-233-0650

Camp Tom-a-Hawk

Darrell Smith
ADA Oklahoma Affiliate
3909 Classen Boulevard, #101
Oklahoma City, OK 73118
405-525-0222

OREGON

Gales Creek Camp

Karen Brown
ADA Oregon Affiliate
6915 SW MacAdam, #130
Portland, OR 97219
503-245-2010

PENNSYLVANIA

Camp Crestfield

Michelle Knight
ADA Pennsylvania Affiliate
5020 Ritter Road, Suite 106
Mechanicsburg, PA 17055
717-691-6170

Camp Setebaid

Michelle Knight
ADA Pennsylvania Affiliate
5020 Ritter Road, Suite 106
Mechanicsburg, PA 17055
717-691-6170

SOUTH CAROLINA

Camp Adam Fisher

Cliff Moore
2200 Green Pines Road
Columbia, SC 29206
803-736-0329

SOUTH DAKOTA

Camp Haunz

Joyce Kaata, RN
1100 S. Euclid
Sioux Falls, SD
57117-5039
605-333-1000;
Beeper 1392

TENNESSEE

Camp Rising Sun

Ben Harrington
American Diabetes
Association
8906 Kingston Pike, 105C
Knoxville, TN 37923
615-531-1129

Camp Sugar Falls

Kristin Robbins
American Diabetes
Association
4205 Hillsboro Road,
Suite 200
Nashville, TN 37215
615-298-3066

Camp Wack-A-Doo

Stephanie Hasenwalder
American Diabetes
Association
317 Oak Street, #103
Chattanooga, TN 37403
615-756-8709

UTAH

Camp Utada

David Okubo, MD
8925 South 2700 West
West Jordan, UT 84088
801-566-9888

VIRGINIA

Camp Holiday Trails

Cleo Velle
PO Box 5806
Charlottesville, VA 22905
804-977-3781

Camp Jordan

Paul Kaplowitz, MD
Department of Pediatrics
MCV Box 140
Richmond, VA
23298-0140
804-786-9616

WASHINGTON

Camp Dudley

Myrl Weaver
Yakima Family YMCA
PO Box 2885
Yakima, WA 98907
509-248-1202

Camp Orkila

Geoff Ball
909 Fourth Avenue
Seattle, WA 98104
206-382-5009

Camp Sealth

Dave Kamenz
Camp Fire
8511 15th Avenue, NE
Seattle, WA 98115
206-461-8550

WYOMING

Camp Hope

Steve and Nancy Johnson
2710 Navarre
Casper, WY 82604
307-265-5865

SOURCES AND REFERENCES

CHAPTER ONE: Fiction Versus Fact

Diabetes Control and Complications Trial (DCCT) funded by the National Institute of Diabetes and Digestive and Kidney Disease. A 10-year research project completed in 1993.

Fund-raising letter, May 17, 1993. Joslin Diabetes Center in Boston, Mass.

Diabetes Forecast. July–August, 1976.

Bradley, Denise J. *Sweet Recovery: A Young Woman's Emotional Ride with Diabetes, Vision Loss, and an Eating Disorder . . . to Health and Freedom,* 1992.

Matthews, L. "Life with Diabetes," *Diabetes Newsletter,* Diabetes Association of Greater Cleveland, 12:2 (April) 1974.

CHAPTER TWO: Basic Questions and Answers on Diabetes

Boshell, B.R. "Fellow Diabetic Is Best Teacher About Regime," *Int. Med. News,* 7:1, No. 10 (May 15), 1974.

Schnatz, J.D. "Self-Care Instruction Reduces Need to Hospitalize Diabetics," *Int. Med. News,* 7:45, No. 17 (Sept. 1), 1974.

Arsham, Gary and Lowe, Ernest. *Diabetes: A Guide to Living Well,* DCI Publishing, 1992.

Duncan, T.G. "Advance for Diabetics—U-100 Insulin Improves Therapy," *Chronic Disease,* 8:1 (Nov.), 1974.

Davidson, J.A.; Galloway, J.A.; Petersen, B.H.; Wentworth, S.M.; and Crabtree, R.E. "Purified Insulins Seen Alleviating Allergies," *Chronic Disease,* 8:1 (Dec.), 1974.

Service, F.J. and Molnar, G.D. "On the Nature of Diabetes and the Need for Urine Testing," *ADA Forecast,* 27:12 (March–April), 1974.

Forsham, P. "Improved Treatment for Diabetes Outlined," *Chronic Disease,* 7:1, No. 11 (Nov.), 1973.

Siperstein, M.D. "Insulin and the Juvenile Diabetic," *Diabetology '74.* Report from the Geigy Symposium, Albuquerque, New Mexico.

Sims, E.A. and Sims, D.F. "A Dialogue about Diabetes and Exercise," *ADA Forecast,* 27:27–31 (Sept.–Oct.), 1974.

CHAPTER THREE: Keeping Control

Diabetes Control and Complications Trial (DCCT) funded by the National Institute of Diabetes and Digestive and Kidney Disease. A 10-year research project completed in 1993.

Gavin II, James, President American Diabetes Association. "Health on Parade," *Parade Magazine,* Nov. 21, 1993.

Gastineau, C.F. "Ask Me Another," *ADA Forecast,* March–April 1973.

CHAPTER FOUR: Food and Drink for the Diabetic

West, K.M. "Diet Therapy of Diabetes: An Analysis of Failure," *Ann. Int. Med.,* 79:425–434 (Sept.), 1973.

French, J.B. "Diabetics Get Dietetic Boost," p. 1C, *The Cleveland Plain Dealer,* Oct. 26, 1974.

Bantle, John P. University of Minnesota Study, 1993.

Brunzell, J.D.; Lerner, R.L.; Prote, D., Jr.; and Bierman, E.L. "Effect of a Fat Free, High Carbohydrate Diet on Diabetic Subjects with Fasting Hyperglycemia," *Diabetes,* 23:138–142 (Feb.), 1974.

Weinsier, R.L.; Seeman, Ann; Herrera, G.; Assal, G.P.; Soeldner, J.S.; and Gleason, R.E. "High-and-Low-Carbohydrate Diets in Diabetes Mellitus: Study on Effects on Diabetic Control, Insulin Secretion, and Blood Lipids," *Ann. Int. Med.,* 80:332–334 (March), 1974.

Davidoff, F.F. *Medical Opinion,* 3:24–30 (June), 1974.

CHAPTER FIVE: Marriage and Children

Beck, P. "Women with Severe Diabetes Advised to Avoid Pregnancy," *Medical Tribune,* p. 29 (Oct. 17), 1973.

"Managing Common Complications in the Newborn," article in *Patient Care,* p.24 (July 1), 1974.

Tyson, J.E.; Khojandi, M.; and Tsai, A.T.M. "Diabetic's Diet Control Key to Normal Birth," *Medical Tribune,* 15:3 (Feb. 20), 1974.

Steel Magnolias, a film based on the play by Richard Harling. 1989.

Rimoin, D.L. "Many Faceted Diabetes is 'A Geneticist's Nightmare'," *Ob. Gyn. News,* p. 20, May 1, 1973.

Pyke, D.A. "Diabetes May Not Be Genetic," *Dimensions,* 2:1 (Nov.), 1973.

Neel, J.V. "Explaining the Genetics Nightmare of Diabetes to Your Patients," *Medical Opinion,* 2:58–68 (Oct.) 1973.

CHAPTER SIX: Complications

Critique of *Counseling and Rehabilitating the Diabetic,* John Cull and Richard Hardy; C.C. Thomas, 1974 (Dolger and Dolger) *ADA Forecast,* 27:13 (Nov.–Dec.), 1974.

Siperstein, M.D. "Aging and Basement Membranes," *Diabetology '74,* Report from Geigy Symposium, Albuquerque, New Mexico.

Black, M.B.; Beck, J.E.; Fridlander, L.S.; Steiner, D.F.; and Rubinstein, A.H. "Diabetic Ketoacidosis Associated with Mumps Infection: Occurrence in a Patient with Macromylasemia," *Ann. Int. Med.,* 78:663–669 (May), 1973.

Moss, J.M. "Current Opinion: Open Letter to *Washington Post,*" *Medical Tribune,* p. 7 (Nov. 13), 1974.

Moss, J.M. and Delawter, D. "Georgetown Study Disputes UGDP Findings," *Int. Med. News,* p. 14 (Oct. 1), 1973.

Kupfer, C. "Evaluation of the Treatment of Diabetic Retinopathy: A Research Project," *The Sight-Saving Review,* pp. 17–28 (Spring), 1973.

O'Grady, G. "Surgery Offers Hope in Diabetic Retinopathy," *Int. Med. News,* 7:23 (Aug.), 1974.

Reinecke, R.D. "New Procedure Aids Blinded Area Diabetic," *Chronic Disease,* 8:23 (Dec.), 1974.

Ellison, J. "Eye Surgery Aids Blinded Area Diabetic," *Cleveland Plain Dealer,* Oct. 9, 1974.

Kussman, M., 35 al. "Early Grafts Urged for Diabetics with Nephropathy," *Medical Tribune,* 15:10, No. 27 (July), 1974.

Hampers, C. "Diabetics Should Not Be Refused Chronic Dialysis," *Int. Med. News,* 7:1 (Sept), 1974.

CHAPTER SEVEN: Diabetes in Children

Harris, W.M. "Teaching the Teacher," *ADA Forecast,* 27:30–32 (Nov.–Dec.), 1974.

Vincent, B. "Juvenile Diabetes: A Tragic Difference in Children," *The Cleveland Press,* May 22, 1974.

Ellison, J. "Premature Aging Linked to Diabetes," *The Cleveland Plain Dealer,* (July 6), 1974.

Rubinstein, A. "Diabetics' Parents Form Foundation," *American Medical News,* p. 8 (Feb. 18), 1974.

Carne, Stuart "How They Treat Diabetes in Children," *Resident and Staff Physician* (July), 1976.

Baker, L.; Bradley, R.F.; Molnar, G.D.; and Knowles, H.C., Jr. "Emotions Called Factor in Instability of Brittle Diabetic," *Int. Med. News,* 7:30–31 (June 1), 1974.

Critique of *Counseling and Rehabilitating the Diabetic* (Dolger and Dolger), *ADA Forecast,* 27:13 (Nov.–Dec.), 1974.

Podoll, E. "Life Style Conflict of the Adolescent Diabetic," *Medical Insight,* pp. 21–26 (March), 1974.

McGraw, R.K. and Travis, L.B. "Psychological Effects of a Special Summer Camp on Juvenile Diabetics, *Diabetes,* 22:275–279 (April), 1973.

Wentworth, S.M. "Diabetic Teens Adventure in Wisconsin Wilderness," *Affiliate Builder,* No. 18:7 (Sept.–Oct.) 1973.

Harris, W.M. Teaching the Teacher," *ADA Forecast,* 27:30–32 (Nov.–Dec.), 1974.

CHAPTER EIGHT: Research on Diabetes

Jackson, Richard A. Pilot Study at Hood Center for Prevention of Childhood Diabetes at Boston's Joslin Diabetes Center, 1989.

Ricketts, H.T. "Pancreatic Transplants: New Wrinkles," *JAMA,* 228: 609–610 (April 29), 1974.

CHAPTER NINE: The Positive Approach

Matthews, L. "Life with Diabetes." *Diabetes Newsletter,* Diabetes Association of Greater Cleveland, 12:2 (April) 1974.

Hill, E. "Life with Diabetes," *Diabetes Newsletter,* Diabetes Association of Greater Cleveland, 12:2 (April), 1974.

Diabetes Forecast, "Diabetes At Home On 'Our House'," (May) 1987.

Talbert, W.F. "40-Love Is Sweeping the Country!" *Prism,* 8:30–35 (Nov.), 1973.

Shaw, J. "Ron Santo and Diabetes: Accept It, Live A Full Life," *Sportsmedicine,* 2:61–63 (June), 1974.

Taylor Bruce: *ADA Forecast* (June–July), 1973.

"Mary Tyler Moore Wins Again," *ADA Forecast,* 27:6 (May–June), 1974.

INDEX

171

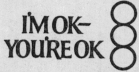

THE NATIONWIDE
#1
BESTSELLER

the
Relaxation
Response

by Herbert Benson, M.D.
with Miriam Z. Klipper

A SIMPLE MEDITATIVE TECHNIQUE
THAT HAS HELPED MILLIONS
TO COPE WITH
FATIGUE, ANXIETY AND STRESS

Available Now—
00676-6/ $5.99 US/ $6.99 Can